When Alzheimer's Touches A Family

A layperson's guide to caring for and understanding the person with Alzheimer's or Dementia

Rebecca Jarrard

Bloomington, IN
authorHOUSE™
Milton Keynes, UK

AuthorHouse™
1663 Liberty Drive, Suite 200
Bloomington, IN 47403
www.authorhouse.com
Phone: 1-800-839-8640

AuthorHouse™ UK Ltd.
500 Avebury Boulevard
Central Milton Keynes, MK9 2BE
www.authorhouse.co.uk
Phone: 08001974150

First published by AuthorHouse 5/15/2006

ISBN: 1-4259-2672-X (sc)

Library of Congress Control Number: 2006903181

Printed in the United States of America
Bloomington, Indiana

This book is printed on acid-free paper.

This book is dedicated to my husband
Dan, who has worked with me,
typing and editing my grammatical errors.
My daughters Salome and Shalamar, who
constantly tell me that they will never
allow me to be placed in a Nursing Home.
Last but not least, all the Alzheimer's and
Dementia patients I have been privileged
to care for during the last seven years.

Pg 93

Contents

Introduction

One day you began to notice subtle changes in the memory of your mother, father, grandmother, or grandfather. You passed it off as their being up in years and this being normal behavior for their age, but you begin to notice that the things they are forgetting are simple, everyday things that they should not be forgetting. You have this frightening, sick feeling in your stomach when you think, "Does my loved one have Alzheimer's?"

This book will help you to understand the disease, its process, how to make sure your loved one gets the care and stimulation he or she needs by you or any facility you may choose to place him or her in.

I believe knowledge is power and the knowledge you gain from this book will give you the power to know what direction to go. It is a resource book that will give you the insight to know how to recognize and deal with the behavioral mood and temperament changes your loved one may go through.

No matter what anyone says, your loved one is unique. Each person enters the Alzheimer's world with his or her unique personality and background. They bring to the disease a part of themselves that is unlike anyone else. Therefore, not all Alzheimer's patients can be treated the same, even though they may exhibit similar symptoms and behaviors.

Much emphasis in the last ten years has been placed in the study of Alzheimer's. While we have come a long way in understanding the disease itself, there is still a need as to understanding how to better care for the person with Alzheimer's.

I personally feel that one of the greatest injustices is placing all stages (early, middle, and late) of Alzheimer's patients in one unit. How cruel for an early stage Alzheimer's patient to be placed with people who are much more confused and volatile than he or she. To daily see people who are much more impaired than themselves can be frightening and can cause them to loose hope and be depressed. This is a form of mental abuse and until families speak up, many Nursing Homes will continue to place all stages of Alzheimer's together and try to care for and treat them all the same.

This book is in two parts. The <u>first</u> will explain the Alzheimer's disease and related Dementia. The <u>second</u> will deal with the care of these fragile people and their behaviors.

As you read, please keep in mind that you have options. There are places (facilities) that will give your loved one a lot of loving care. It may take work to find one, but you don't want to just settle for anything. I feel sure you will find that special place that recognizes your loved one as a unique and special person, just as you believe he or she is.

There are many privately owned Nursing Homes and Assisted Living Facilities in the United States. I was privileged to have worked in one owned by the Hovnanian family. Their desire to make life as enjoyable as possible for people with Dementia and Alzheimer's is exemplary. Unlike most owners of Long-term Care Facilities, the Hovnanian family saw the need to have a separate unit for each stage of the Alzheimer's disease; therefore we had a memory impaired assisted living, a second stage and an end stage unit. The staff on all these units is specifically trained to care for the stage with which they work.

There are places like the Haven that are owned by genuinely caring people who have the utmost respect for the elderly, especially when they have a mentally debilitating disease such as Alzheimer's and Dementia, that makes them vulnerable to caregivers. On a daily basis, respect, privacy, independence, and autonomy was encouraged as we worked with the mentally impaired who were entrusted to our care.

This book would not have been possible without the time I spent as the Director and Wellness Nurse on the Haven, in Brick, New Jersey. When the Haven is mentioned throughout this book, it is referring to a 30-bed memory impaired unit. All the residents had a diagnosis of Alzheimer's or Dementia.

I would also like to acknowledge the teaching that Dr. Paul Bryman gave me. He served as the main Physician I worked with on the Haven. Without his helping me to understand the disease and how it affects people, I could have never done the job as I did. He helped me to enable my patients to have as much quality of life as possible and for that I will always be grateful.

If you have a loved one with Alzheimer's or Dementia, this book has been written for you. It is a practical, user friendly guide to assist you in understanding and caring for your loved one.

I utilized all the care techniques you will read about in this book. My staff was trained to employ these techniques as well. Going to seminars and training sessions – learning all these techniques gave me a desire to share what I had learned with you. My hope is that, with this book as a help, you will better understand the disease of Alzheimer's/Dementia; and therefore be made capable to give the right kind of compassionate care. And when you do have to place your loved one in a Long-term Care Facility, you will have some tools to enable you to choose the best possible facility for not only your loved one, but also to give you the peace of mind you deserve.

I have kept everything you read as simple as possible. Let me reiterate – this is a layman's guide to Alzheimer's and Dementia, NOT a medical book. If you do not understand what you are reading, it will not help you.

As you read, you may see many behavior patterns in your loved one that I share in the book. Also, you will read stories and see parts of your situation with your family member in them.

As you read, you will also discover repetition in this book, but one of the best ways to learn is through repetition.

A Quick Reference Of Terms And Definitions Related To Alzheimer's

As a general rule, a "Glossary Of Terms And Definitions" is placed at the end of a book. However, I am placing it at the beginning of this book. These are terms of a technical, medical nature and I have endeavored, in the spirit and intent of this book, to explain them in practical language so as to assist you in better understanding what you are about to read.

Abandon: The patient feels like a child – frightened and alone – when the person with whom the Alzheimer's patient is most familiar leaves.

ADL: This is an acronym for "Activities of Daily Living." These include dressing, bathing, activities, etc.

Aphasia: When the patient can no longer give an appropriate verbal response.

Assisted Living. Where people go when they are not sick or debilitated to the point of needing nursing care around the clock. They just need a minimal amount of assistance.

Autonomy: The ability to make decisions and choices that relate to oneself.

Behavior: The way a person acts or reacts.

Catastrophic reaction: When a person with Alzheimer's reacts to simple stimuli with screaming, combativeness, or extremely angry words.

Cat Scan: A radiological test that is used oftentimes to diagnose Dementia that has been caused by a stroke or head trauma.

Cognitive: The ability to make safe, sensible, rational decisions.

Combativeness: When a patient reacts physically to stimuli, such as trying to hit or bite someone who is trying to give them a shower.

Dehydration: When a person's body fluid level is dangerously low.

Delusions: When the confused patient sees or hears things that are not there.

Dementia: When brain cells shrink or die, and the patient's cognitive abilities are impaired.

Failure to thrive: When a person does not eat enough to sustain life.

Finger Painting: When a confused person smears feces on walls, furniture, etc.

Hospice: An organization of specially trained Nurses that works with patients who have an end-stage disease so as to make the dying process as easy as possible for both the patient and family members.

Hypercelcemia: Too much calcium in the blood. This can cause confusion and Dementia-like symptoms. *Pg. 58*

Hyperchondriosis: When a person with Temperal Lobe Dementia fixates on one disease and they believe they are dying from that disease.

Hypersensitivity: When senses such as taste, touch, and hearing are heightened. The patient may not like being touched or may be just the opposite – such as touching people's hair, clothes or hands.

Hypochondriac: A person who picks up on other people's illnesses and believes that they have the symptoms of those illnesses.

Hyposensitivity: When the senses of touch, hearing, taste, etc. are lowered. The patient may not respond to touch, may not hear well, and response may be diminished.

Hypothyroidism: A decrease of production of the thyroid gland. A low thyroxin level can cause confusion.

Impulsive: Making quick decisions and acting on them without thinking of consequences.

Long-term Care: Generally refers to a Nursing Home. People who are physically debilitated and the family cannot care for them nor can the patients care for themselves usually go to a Nursing Home where they have nursing care 24 hours a day.

Loved one, resident, patient: All refer to the individual with Alzheimer's or Dementia who lives at home, a Nursing Home, or Assisted Living Facility.

Medical Director: A Physician who sits on the Board of a Nursing Home and assists in making policy and procedures relating to the medical care of the residents.

Modeling: When you act out what you want your loved one to do, such as brushing your teeth to show them how to brush theirs.

Motor skills: Walking, using the hands and arms.

Neurosyphilis: Syphilis of the brain that leads to Dementia.

Paranoia: When the patient feels someone is out to get him or her or take what they have, such as their money.

Podiatrist: A Doctor who specializes in the care of the foot.

Reminiscing: Going back, through the use of pictures, stories, etc., in the lives of the patient with Alzheimer's to a time when he or she was young.

Shuffling: When the part of the brain that controls motor skills is damaged and the patient does not pick the feet up, but somewhat rubs them on the floor when walking.

Staging: The degrees that Alzheimer's begins and ends with.
Stage I – Mild
Stage II – Moderate

Stage III – Severe
Stage IV – End

Stimuli: Anything that creates a reaction.

Sundowners: Occurs in confused people, usually between the hours of 3-5 p.m. They get more confused and can exhibit agitated behavior.

Transition: When a person with Alzheimer's advances to another stage of the disease.

UTI: Urinary tract infection. A urine test and blood work will reveal this.

Wandering: When a patient with Alzheimer's continually walks and does not want to sit down.

Chapter One

What Alzheimer's Is

Alzheimer's is a form of Dementia – the most common type. Not all Dementia patients have Alzheimer's, but all Alzheimer's patients have Dementia. The length of the Alzheimer's disease is 8-12 years, and has affected approximately 4 million people in the United States.

Alzheimer's has two major forms: early onset and normal onset. It is a terminal disease. There is no cure. Alzheimer's is an irreversible and progressive disease that destroys memory, thinking skills and eventually causes the patient not to be able to carry out the most simple of tasks. Its symptoms are generally predictable with individual variation.

Alzheimer's derives its name from a German Physician, Alois Alzheimer, who first identified the Alzheimer's condition in 1906, when he performed an autopsy on the brain of a woman who had severe memory loss. Dr. Alzheimer noted plaques and tangles in the patient's brain and thus concluded that because of these findings the woman could not remember everyday things and could not follow through on simple tasks. These plaques are clumps of protein that accumulate outside the brain's nerve cells. Tangles are twisted strands of another protein that form inside the brain's cells. Because of these plaques and tangles, the brain has a disruption in the transmission of information – new information is not retained.

Alzheimer's cannot be 100 % accurately diagnosed, but with a good physical exam and mental work-up, it can be diagnosed with a very high percentage of accuracy – approximately 90%.

I have told families to think of a spider web hanging between two small trees. The web is perfect in its design. This represents a healthy brain. I then tell them to take a hand and go to the middle of the spider web and pull it toward them slightly and let it go. Now you have a brain that has been besieged by Alzheimer's.

The brain with Alzheimer's shrinks to 1/3 its original size, so you can see that with the actual loss/death of brain cells, the ability to function in a normal way is not possible. Therefore, your responsibility, above all else, is to keep the loved one safe.

Early in the disease the Alzheimer's patient looses ¼ of his or her words. Later they miss ½ of their words. They reach a point where they read your body language more than understand your words. This is why, when we speak to them, we look directly at them and speak slowly, in short sentences and in a normal tone if they have no hearing loss. If you are angry and you approach them, they may think you are angry with them – so approach them calmly and treat them gently. This will aid in their remaining calm when you are trying to give them directions.

They may be able to recall in detail memories from 50 years ago, but not recall anything from yesterday or earlier today. They may have emotional memories and when they do, it may be as if the death of a loved one just happened today. The Alzheimer's patient may remember familiar faces and places. They may be able to chat even though they cannot go into detail.

People with Alzheimer's tend to typically develop a loss of speech or use unfamiliar words, behavior, and routine. Some abilities are lost but others may be retained.

Skills and abilities typically LOST are:

<u>Memory skills</u>. Involves immediate recall, short-term memory, categorical information, and clarity of time and place.

<u>Language skills</u>. Descriptive words, reading comprehension, spoken communicative words, socially accepted expressions of emotions, the ability to express needs and desires.

<u>Motor skills</u>. Getting started, non-completion of tasks, cannot organize, loss of visual field, hyposensitivity to touch, sound, light, etc., or a hypersensitivity to these things (see Glossary).

<u>Emotional impulse and control skills</u>. No longer can demand respect although they still want it. Loss of emotional control, loss of control of speech, using language that is inappropriate, loss of control of impulsive actions, loss of the ability to keep private thoughts and actions in private places.

On the other side of the coin, skills and abilities that are RETAINED are:

<u>Memory skills</u>. Emotional memories such as marriage, birth of children, death of a close relative, memories from many years ago, making up stories, procedural memories (routines).

<u>Language use skills</u>. Desire to communicate (using their hands or actions to describe), reading out loud, following a rhythm of speech, music and song (such as big band presentations), automatic speech, cursing or using sex words (saying extremely vulgar words), non-verbal communication of needs and wants.

<u>Motor skills</u>. Movement patterns for pieces of tasks, can do the mechanics but not well, looks for things, recognizes familiar faces and voices.

<u>Emotional and impulse control skills</u>. Desire to be respected, say what they think although not cor-rectly, ability to feel emotions and have needs, do

what you want to, sometimes feel badly after bad behavior or saying inappropriate things, sometimes behaving in public if reminded by the person they are with.

With the loss of so much, you can see that your loved one is doing the best he or she can with what brain tissue is present. You are the "normal" one. If change is necessary, you have to do it. Your loved one is no longer capable of changing. Their brains are sick. Just as you would not yell at a heart to beat correctly or for it to be normal, you should not yell at the Alzheimer's patient when he or she is not acting normal. Their brains are sick and they need the same gentle, loving care as the patient with any other physical disease.

Chapter Two

Early Signs Of
Alzheimer's

There are early signs that can alert you to the possibility that your loved one may be developing Alzheimer's. These are listed and explained so as to share with you knowledge that will assist in your getting help for your loved one as early as possible.

First and foremost, there is memory loss of recently learned information, such as telephone numbers and names. Sometimes they forget their own addresses.

Second, difficulty performing familiar tasks. Because of the loss of executive functioning tasks that are simple, everyday tasks are difficult to follow through. Steps may be skipped; the task may be started but simply abandoned due to the patient not knowing what to do next. An Alzheimer's patient may no longer know the steps to cooking a familiar meal, how to use a stove or participate in simple hobbies such as sewing, painting, etc. They may not even know what a telephone is for or call numbers they do not know, thinking they are calling a daughter or son. They may call the correct number, but not know why they called.

Third, there may be definite changes in personality. The quiet mom, dad, sister or aunt may become very vocal and inappropriate with language, using profanity. An independent person may become very fearful and dependent on a particular family member.

<u>Fourth</u>, there may be dramatic mood changes, such as going from tears to anger to aggression – and this can happen very quickly. Within minutes a patient may not remember these mood swings and then often wonder why they are being confronted about previous actions. A person who is generally calm may become extremely agitated and actually become combative, and moments later have no memory of the actions. If these actions are brought on by a disagreement with your loved one, remember it is not important for you to be right. They will not remember whether you are right or wrong. Make it easier for you both – don't argue with them. The person you knew is slowly, but surely slipping away from self, you, and others before your very eyes.

<u>Fifth</u>, there may be a loss of initiative or desire to do everyday things such as housework, yard work, or going out to dinner. Simple tasks may tire them. They may be very passive, sleep more, and watch more television. This is a difficult thing to watch if your loved one was always active and involved. If he or she was a positive person, he or she may become negative.

Sixth, the person with early Alzheimer's may forget familiar places and how to perform familiar tasks. They may get disoriented on their own block or street. They can even get lost in their own home. They may tell you that the room they are in is not a part of their home and possibly become very agitated if they cannot get out, if they believe they are in the wrong house. They may put something on the stove, lay down and forget they have turned the stove on. This is a very dangerous thing. People have actually been killed in house fires by turning on a stove and then forgetting to turn it off. Some Alzheimer's patients have wandered off and gotten lost in wooded areas and died because they became disoriented and were exposed to the elements.

Seventh, there may be compromised judgment. At best, their judgment is compromised. They may not put on a coat to go outside, may put on 3 or 4 shirts, several pairs of pants, wear soiled clothing, not want to bath or shave, hair gets oily and stringy because they no longer can take a bath. They cannot follow the steps to bathing or taking a shower. They may be fearful of water and even a shiny floor may be perceived as water. Money looses its value to the Alzheimer's patient. They may pay extreme amounts of money for people to do simple tasks for them. I had a friend whose family told me that a loved one with Alzheimer's had paid a teenage boy $100.00 several times to take her to the drug store which was only 2 blocks away. (If your loved one lives alone and your visits are infrequent this could happen. There are people who will definitely exploit the aged). She also went to the bank and withdrew almost $6,000.00 and lost it. She had no memory of any of this when her family inquired where the money was. I had an aunt who bought thousands of dollars worth of merchandise from "telemarketers" and when she died, hundreds of boxes were in her home, unopened. When simple home repairs are needed, the early Alzheimer's patient may pay extremely large amounts of money to have these repairs done. Remember that money has little or no value to them.

Eighth, abstract thinking may become adversely affected. Numbers become very difficult to work with. They can no longer balance a checkbook, cannot write out checks or add and subtract simple math problems. Some Alzheimer's patients forget numbers entirely.

Ninth, a very common problem the early Alzheimer's patient has is misplacing things, putting things in unusual places such as: their purse in the refrigerator or milk in the pantry cabinet. Shoes, clothes, and purses have been found in refrigerators. They may be cleaning and putting things away, and to them this is the appropriate place. During this period the Alzheimer's patient may become very paranoid – accusing loved ones or caregivers of stealing things that they have put away, but cannot remember where. Money can become a large, delicate, and sometimes confrontational issue; the Alzheimer's patient may hide money and then swear it was stolen. If you are the caregiver, you may be the one accused. If this happens offer to help look for it. Do not argue - it will be futile.

<u>Tenth</u>, a problem with language may develop. The Alzheimer's patient may not be able to say certain words. They may loose the ability to write. They may start a sentence and forget to finish it or make up words. I had a patient once who told me, as her husband was leaving the room, that "he is going to the corner to watch the turkles go by." If the Alzheimer's patient wants to wash his or her face, they may ask for "that thing" (referring to a wash cloth) to wash the face. Remember, here again, that if your loved one lives alone and your visits are infrequent, you may not realize how your loved one has advanced in the disease process. The higher functioning and the more visible your loved one is to you, a caregiver, or friends, the quicker someone will notice that things are just not right. The more alone they are and the less social they are, the easier it is for them to get into situations where

they are exploited or placed in harm's way. If you visit a relative and you notice even subtle changes, you should take action to make sure someone you trust will check on them and get them into a safe environment before they are harmed in their home or by someone outside the home. If a stranger begins to take interest in a confused, elderly loved one - beware! Find out as much as possible about the stranger and also do an inventory to make sure valuable items are not missing. You might even have to remove valuables from the home because your loved one with Alzheimer's may give them away to total strangers.

If you have a loved one that has Alzheimer's, you can relate to many of these symptoms. You have probably come to realize that each day there is a little more loss of the person you have known. This is a very sad disease – not only to the patient, but also for you as the family. You must realize that this is a disease. The changes in personality, mood swings, accusing, cursing, etc. are coming from a very sick loved one. This is not your family member, as you knew him or her. These outrageous things are not being done with any malice or intent. They have lost the ability to control their thought processes or their response to situations. Just as a patient with congestive heart failure will grow weaker and weaker from the fluid build-up in the body, the Alzheimer's patient will grow weaker and weaker in what they are capable of doing, because of the Alzheimer's disease process.

Since the process cannot be stopped, it is your responsibility to protect and care for your loved one to the best of your ability so that they can have as happy and safe a life as possible, while trying to live with this horrible disease. Your commitment, patience, and care will be an invaluable gift to your loved one. They may never be able to say "thank you," but when all is said and done, you will have the peace of mind in knowing you have done everything in your power to give your loved one the quality of life they deserve in their final years.

I have a friend who recently lost her husband to this disease. For the last three years of his life he was completely bed bound. She saw each day that he was cared for – kept clean, turned, and given nourishment. At the time of his death she was on the bed, right by his side. This lady is grieving, and her grief is borne out of genuine sorrow for the loss of her precious husband. She has no "guilt grief," which is a grief many people experience. This is a gift she has given herself because of the vigilance she invested in the care of her husband. He died in a Nursing Home, but she did not put him there and forget him. She remained a vital part of his care until the moment he died.

Chapter Three

Staging Alzheimer's

Whenever you take your loved one to his or her family physician and the Doctor suspects they may have the early signs and symptoms of Alzheimer's, he or she may be referred to a Neurologist, a Psychiatrist, or a Physician that is specialized in Alzheimer's and related Dementia. When this occurs, the Doctor you see will do an extensive exam. This is a test that will define short-term memory loss. The questions are usually easily answered by a well mind, but if your loved one has Alzheimer's the questions are difficult. The test may include such questions as: "What is your whole name? When is your birthday? What is today's date? Who is the President of the United States? Who was the previous President?" The test may also consist of asking the individual to name three objects such as an apple, a penny, and a pencil. The Doctor will ask a few more questions and then ask your loved one to recall the three objects mentioned above. They may be asked to name their children and grandchildren. This may indeed be difficult if they do in fact have Alzheimer's.

After this mental exam, along with a physical exam and blood work, the Doctor may stage your loved one's Alzheimer's after all the tests are completed and reviewed. Some of the areas for testing include folate, B-12, thyroid, a test for syphilis, and a few other tests that can rule out a chemical imbalance that could be causing Alzheimer-like symptoms.

Generally, there are three stages of classification for Alzheimer's: Mild, Moderate, and Severe. But there is a fourth stage that will be discussed as well.

In the **<u>Mild or Early Stage of Alzheimer's</u>** the patient may not show a lot of definitive symptoms. The higher functioning ability the person has had, the quicker we notice subtle changes. If your father or mother or aunt is a CPA or banker, and he or she begins to have trouble with numbers or if they are a librarian or teacher and have difficulty reading, you notice right away that something is wrong. But if your loved one never finished grammar school, cannot read or write very well, you may not notice the very early signs of Alzheimer's as readily. So as we look at Stage One or Mild Alzheimer's, try to keep this in mind.

The Mild Stage of Alzheimer's can last from two to four years. Family members or the patients themselves may be the only ones to notice the changes. They may say, "It seems lately I cannot remember anything," or a family member may jokingly say, "Mom, it seems lately that you can't remember anything. Don't you think you should be checked for Alzheimer's?" Everyone laughs, but if mom has, in actuality thought that she might have the early signs of Alzheimer's, this can be a frightening situation for her.

The symptoms of this phase are repetitive questions. My grandmother had Alzheimer's and she would ask the same question over and over when I visited. She would ask such things as: "are you married, do you have children, how old are you, where do you live?" Then the cycle would start over.

Short-term memory loss is failing to remember where things are placed (like a purse, a piece of clothing, etc.), forgetting names of friends they have known for years, relatives and familiar objects. They may not know what a certain kitchen appliance is for, or not be able to turn on the television or radio because they do not know the functions of the buttons. They may get in their car and not know where the keys go.

There may also be personality changes. The person that was the life of the party becomes passive and quiet, shows little expression; or the quiet, reserved person may become agitated, scream at people and children. There may also be disorientation which is displayed by going to appointments on the wrong days or at the wrong times – they may not be able to tell time or understand the significance of time.

The early Alzheimer's patient may lose interest in things that they once took a lot of care and interest in, such as: cleanliness of their surrounding, keeping their hair and nails clean and presentable, making sure that the wardrobe coordinated - all the way to matching shoes and jewelry. With Alzheimer's they may put on several layers of clothes or not wear appropriate clothing for various settings or occasions. They may go for days and not bath, wash, or comb their hair. They do not see this as abnormal behavior. They may come into the living room with no clothes on at all. To them this is not an attempt to be an exhibitionist or embarrass anyone – this is the result of a very debilitating disease. They do not see the right or wrong of this action - they just do it.

<u>The Second Stage or Moderate Stage of Alzheimer's</u> is characterized by increased confusion, especially about recent things, an increase of anxiety or depression, speech may not make a lot of sense, sentences are incomplete, may be argumentative and have extreme mood changes.

Recently a gentleman told me about his father arguing with him over some insignificant thing and his dad became so agitated that he threw his coffee cup at the son. This was frightening to the son, as he had never seen his dad like that before.

In the Moderate Stage, the person with Alzheimer's may get lost easily. They can actually get lost in their own home and not recognize familiar surroundings. They may try to get out because they think they are in someone else's house. If they get out they may not recognize their neighborhood. The memory is seriously impaired. In this stage they may not realize they have a memory problem and feel perfectly normal.

Behavioral problems may become greater and the patient more difficult to handle. The individual may be combative and in this phase they must be protected from themselves and the caregiver must also be protected. They may wander more, not being able to sit for long periods of time. They may walk in circles or throughout the house looking in closets as if they do not recognize where they are. They are not familiar with the home they have lived in for years – one room is no different than another. This can be a dangerous stage because if they get out of the house they can walk for hours and not know where they are or where they are going. They may have difficulty sleeping – up and down all during the night. They may also become incontinent of urine and feces. They may urinate in plants, corners or on the bathroom floor. They may have a bowel movement in the middle of the floor; or soil themselves and in an effort to clean themselves, put feces on the floor, walls, mirrors, or in dresser drawer (this is referred to as finger painting).

The Alzheimer's person may become very impulsive during this stage as depicted in such things as: putting an empty pan on the hot stove burner and then walking out of the kitchen; taking everything out of the refrigerator and placing it on the counter; taking their clothes out of the closet and off the hangers; putting objects in the wrong place such as a shoe in the refrigerator. This is bazaar behavior for sure, but this is the result of a very sick and confused mind.

The Third Stage is the Severe Stage of Alzheimer's, and is without a doubt one of the more difficult stages for the family members. This stage goes from 3 years until death and carries with it severe confusion and disorientation. The wandering is worsened, motor skills are impaired, there is difficulty walking and there may even be difficulties in swallowing. There may be an increase in agitation and the inability to follow simple commands. They cannot care for themselves. If they are not fed, they simply do not eat. They have lost the ability to cook for themselves. They may go for weeks without bathing, brushing their teeth and will fight anyone who tries to give them a bath. Physically they are at a greater risk of infections, especially if they are diabetic. They are not clean and urinary tract infections are common. Sometimes they can get very sick before this is noticed, because they cannot communicate pain or abnormal drainage from sores to their families. At this stage, if the loved one is still at home, he or she must be assessed by the caregiver routinely to prevent illness.

I cared for a lady in this phase of the disease and she was probably one of the more severe wanderers I ever saw. She would walk until she simply could not take another step. If we tried to get her to sit, she became combative. The only thing we could do was to see that all her basic needs were met. If she was walking during a meal, we saved her meal and fed her when she sat down. We totally reworked our schedule relative to her, around her wandering. Eventually, she ceased her wandering and it came to the place and time when we had to lead her to everything – meals, activities, and showers. She was no longer combative, but very childlike – having to be given total care. She no longer had the ability to make choices of any kind.

Let me share with you here that if your loved one gets more agitated or confused than usual, get him or her to a Doctor. They may have a urinary tract infection or be getting dehydrated.

Stage Four. At this stage, TOTAL supervision and care is necessary. The patient cannot understand when he or she is talked to. They no longer can remember how to read. They forget their children's names and faces. They even forget themselves in this stage. I once had a patient who came out of her room frightened and crying. I asked what was wrong and she tried to tell me that someone was in her room. Holding onto my sweater, she led me back to her room and right away I knew that she thought someone was inside. One of my Aides and I went into the room with her and we looked in the closet, under the bed and behind the door, but no one was there. We went into the bathroom and as she passed the mirror she huddled against me. When she saw her reflection in the mirror she grabbed me very tightly. I knew she was frightened. She was the stranger in the room - she did not remember what she looked like and her own reflection was a stranger looking back at her.

During this stage, the Alzheimer's patient may develop a "failure to thrive syndrome." They don't eat enough to sustain life. They may have to be given supplements such as Ensure, high calorie cookies or foods. Dehydration is a diagnosis that is common during this stage. Dehydration can throw the patient into a very sick state and can lead to kidney failure and an electrolyte imbalance. Fluids should be offered and encouraged regularly. Sometimes a feeding tube is placed to maintain the body's balance and to keep the patient from starving to death.

In this stage many families allow the disease to follow it's natural progression and the patient dies, but some families choose to keep their loved ones alive as long as possible. A lot of ethical questions are dealt with among families during this time. It is during this time that a family is either brought closer or oftentimes, because of disagreements over the kind of care that is desired for the loved one, a family is split and hard feelings are formed. It is very sad when this happens because if the loved one that is being fought over could understand what was taking place, he or she would be heartbroken at these unproductive disputes.

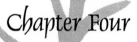

Chapter Four

Behavior Of The
Alzheimer's Patient

Behaviors of an Alzheimer's patient can cause havoc in a family. Alzheimer's patients can have such temperament changes that bring about bazaar behaviors. If this chapter helps you in any way, it should be to cause you to become angry – angry at the disease, but love with everything in you the person with Alzheimer's.

When we are angry at the disease, we will be driven to know more about it and seek to understand it more fully. We will know that the negative behaviors are a result of the disease and that your loved one is simply a conduit of these behaviors. In their normal state of mind they would not be this way.

When caregivers forget who is the real enemy of the Alzheimer's patient, they often attack the patient, sometimes physically – sometimes verbally – sometimes emotionally. The enemy is the Alzheimer's disease – NOT your loved lone.

Behavior can change quickly when there is a destruction of brain cells. Normally, we are capable of making choices and decisions that keep us safe, but when Alzheimer's patients find themselves in frightening, vulnerable situations, they may react in extremely dangerous or inappropriate ways.

This behavior is usually not comfortable for the caregiver, but it also is not comfortable for patients either. As a caregiver you can make these negative or challenging behaviors less of a problem by knowing what contributes to the behavior and minimize these things. Then the problems they cause will also be minimized. You may discover that, as the caregiver, you will have to make many choices and decisions for them in order for them to remain physically healthy and safe.

Some of the most prevalent behaviors that present a challenge to caregivers are: wandering, paranoia, depression, agitation and aggression, repetitive actions, sleep disturbance, and sexual inappropriateness. Not all patients will exemplify the same behaviors. Oftentimes the behavior is the patient's way of communicating discomfort or displeasure. The resident or patient may be tired, hurting, or hungry, but cannot say the words to let you know they have these needs. So your challenge as a caregiver is to find out what the behavior is trying to say. Some behaviors cannot be explained. I know a pastor's wife who has a sister with Alzheimer's. Her sister went to the yard, dug up the plants, brought them into the house and placed them on the dining room table.

<u>Wandering</u>. What causes wandering in the patient with Dementia? Some of the more common reasons a patient wanders are confusion, restlessness, fear, stress, unmet needs, medication, or past behavior. The very first thing I want to say about the wanderer is that the area in which they wander

must be kept safe and hazard free. The confused patient cannot think quickly enough to side step or step over something in the path. The path must be kept clean of obstacles that can cause them to trip and fall. Having said that, we will discuss in detail the causes of wandering.

A. Confusion. People with Alzheimer's often wander because they are confused as to the time. The patient may believe it is the year, 1930, when he or she was a child, and they are walking to their grandmother's house. They may be walking home from school.

B. Fear. Residents may wander when they are fearful, thinking they are getting away from a dangerous situation or a person of whom they are afraid.

C. Restlessness. Some residents wander when they feel bored or restless; they become a seeker – trying to find something. This is why it is so important for the Long-term Care Facility in which you place your loved one to have a good activities department.

D. Stress. The resident may be trying to get away from a stressful situation such as someone else screaming or being combative, or an extremely loud or active activity.

E. Medication. This can sometimes increase the patient's level of confusion and restlessness. I have seen this happen with many of my Alzheimer's patients when the Doctor was trying to find the right medication or the right amount of medication.

F. Past Behavior. They may be going to work, looking for an old friend or they need to help a past family member. I had a patient that was an attorney and he was constantly asking me to let him out to go to his office or to go to the courthouse. Because of this, he wandered throughout the unit, trying to find a door that would open.

G. Unmet Basic Needs (such as being hungry, thirsty, or needing to go to the bathroom). These basic needs will cause the patient to go searching – trying to find water or food. It is important to offer "toileting" every couple of hours throughout the day.

Wandering may not be completely bad – it can have benefits. Yes, the caregiver must always remember, whether in the home or in a facility, that the resident who wanders may fall or wander outside and get lost; but the wandering can also improve mobility, circulation, and increase the appetite.

Paranoia. When a person is suspicious or mistrusting of others. This is not based on fact, but the patient may accuse loved ones of stealing from them or caregivers of taking things that they have actually misplaced. I have had patients to get extremely agitated, thinking someone had taken their jewelry, but upon a complete search, we would find the items in a coat pocket, a drawer, or maybe in a suit case or even in the refrigerator in their room. The patient may also accuse a spouse of being unfaithful.

Some of the causes of paranoia are: lack of sensory stimulation, memory loss, medication and side effects from some illnesses such as dehydration, anemia or infection. If the patient suddenly becomes paranoid or suspicious, the Doctor may need to do some blood work to rule out anemia or dehydration. Medications should be looked at to see if the patient is taking something new that might cause this behavior. If a patient is left alone, he or she may be afraid and due to the lack of sensory stimulation may become suspicious of people. I admitted several people who had lived alone for years and they were paranoid or suspicious of others. Fortunately, with the correct medication, their paranoia disappeared.

If your loved one is exhibiting paranoia or suspicious behavior, it is extremely important that you find a Doctor that knows how to deal with the various types of Dementia. In another section of this book we will notice and deal with various types of Dementia.

Depression. This is a disorder of the brain that can cause extreme feelings of sadness and helplessness. The more prominent characteristics of depression are: sadness, crying, withdrawal from others and activities, fearfulness, sleeping problems and a loss of appetite. Most Alzheimer's/Dementia patients exhibit, at sometime or the other, depression. Treatment is very important and a lot of people respond well.

Some of the causes of depression are a chemical imbalance in the brain and stress. This is not only the cause of depression in the elderly, but for all people who are depressed. Alzheimer's, due to the very nature of the disease, causes a chemical imbalance in the brain. The older population is under more stress today with financial instability and health care costing so much. The older generation is stressed over their money running out before they do.

Medical intervention is extremely important for your loved one when signs of depression appear. If they are sad, not eating, loosing that gleam in their eyes or no longer show excitement over exciting things, get medical help. The right medication could very well make their life and yours much better. Depression is common in the earlier stages of Alzheimer's. People are still pretty much with it, but are beginning to realize that there are some things just not right with them. They may come to believe in their aware times that they might have Alzheimer's so you can see how easily this could cause them to become depressed. The earlier they can get on the right anti-depressant, the better off they will be.

You, as a caregiver, can help by also keeping the patient busy with activities they enjoy. Talk about enjoyable memories, such as their children or their childhood, be positive with them and smile while around them, and encourage them to go outside in the sunshine on sunny days. Take them for drives in their old neighborhoods and reminisce with them. All these things can be helpful. It is important that during these times of depression you are supportive and the person with Alzheimer's is not left alone throughout the day. Activity, Activity, Activity – is an important key in helping the early Alzheimer's patient with depression.

<u>Agitation and Aggression</u>. These are two behavior changes that often times occur with the Alzheimer's patient and are difficult behaviors for family members and caregivers to have to deal with. It is during this time that Alzheimer's patients can become dangerous to themselves as well as others. Agitation is an expression of distress. Aggression is a hostile feeling or action that can be in the form of physical abuse or verbal abuse. Some of the causes for agitation and aggression are pain, rejection, loss, frustration, a perceived threat, an attempt to keep or obtain a possession, wrong ap-

proach by another patient or caregiver, and over-stimulation.

I won't go into a lengthy discussion about all of these things that can trigger an act of aggression or make a patient agitated, but I will share a story to show how easily an act of aggression can come about in a given situation.

One of the gentlemen on my Alzheimer's unit had gone out to eat with his daughter and upon leaving the restaurant, her dad picked up a handful of matches and put them in his pocket. The daughter saw this and tried to get him to give them to her, but he refused – cursing at her in the restaurant. When he returned to the unit, she informed me that her dad had the matches in his pocket. This gentleman had smoked a pipe for years and to him, the matches he had taken were for his pipe; but there was no smoking on the unit (we took the patients outside if they had a desire to smoke). I knew he would get extremely agitated and aggressive, both verbally and physically, if I tried to take the matches from him so I went to my office, got a candle, and asked the patient if I could borrow a match to light it. He said, "Sure," and gave me a pack of the matches. There were four more packs in his pocket. Later that day I went into his room and borrowed the matches again, upon which he gave me the second book of matches. This happened four times and he had one pack left. I suggested to my staff that they ask him, when they got him ready for bed, to place the matches by his pipe so he would know where they were. This he did, and during the night they took the matches. We kept a close eye on him while he had the matches in his possession, but a very difficult situation was averted by my patiently taking the matches from him. It took longer, but the outcome was better because this particular resident could get very agitated and aggressive with staff if he felt the least bit threatened. He was a very strong willed – generally angry man.

Sometimes it takes a lot of thought and patience to acquire a desired result, but quick or impulsive reactions can cause a patient to hurt you as a caregiver or you to hurt them.

Some of the more extreme behaviors related to aggression are biting, hitting, kicking, pinching, pushing, threatening, cursing, and name-calling. When your loved one shows these behaviors it is important for you to know it is the disease acting out – not your loved one.

If you notice a frown on your loved one's face, he or she is pacing, talking loudly, shaking door knobs, shaking fists at you, trying to get a locked door open, screams, acting hostile or they are unable to rest, try to find out what is causing the agitation. If you cannot find out what is the cause, the best thing for you to do is back off – don't argue, don't yell or talk loudly to them, don't get aggressive with them (this happens all too often). Don't take their aggression personally. This may indeed be difficult for you if you are a spouse, daughter or son, but offer encouragement and remember this anger is not with you. Don't scold the person or use force to make him or her to do tasks. Don't intimidate your love one or restrain him or her. Don't back them into a corner and have other members of the family crowd around them. This will be extremely traumatic.

There are things you can do to help your loved one through these periods of agitation and aggression. Try to find out the cause, be supportive, use distraction, try to get them away from the situation that is causing their agitation, be respectful (say, "please, thank you"). Try not to become angry, turn off loud noises and of utmost importance, do everything possible to keep your loved one and yourself out of harm's way. Don't let them hurt you. They will not hurt you on purpose, but they may accidentally hurt you by throwing something, hitting you, pushing you, or striking at you with a cane or walker. Remember that they can be dangerous during these periods of the Alzheimer's disease and that it is the disease acting out - not your loved one.

There is one more behavior that often times carries with it extreme agitation and this is Sundowner's Syndrome; so named because of the behavior changes that occur late in the afternoon, as the sun goes down. It could be the result of the patient being tired and cannot process things as well as during the day. The best way to deal with Sundowner's Syndrome is by closing curtains, turning on a lot of lights, having calming activities and make sure basic needs are met (the patient is fed, has plenty of fluids and has been "toileted"). You may find that you will have to become the expert at redirecting during this period.

Repetitive actions. This is when the person does a specific thing over and over again. I had a resident who folded her clothes and placed them in her chest drawers continually when she was in her room. Some people will say the same thing over and over, such as "Can I go home?" or "Have you seen my mother?"

For people who exhibit repetitive behavior, redirection is one of the best ways to deal with them. Try to get them doing something else. For example, the lady who repeatedly folded her clothes was kept out of her room as much as possible and involved in as many activities as possible. For the resident who continually asked about her mother, we showed her pictures of her mom and reminisced with her. If you try to take things out of their hands that they are being repetitive with, they could very well become frustrated and agitated. If you say to someone who is asking repeatedly where his or her mother is: "You know your mother died," or "Your mother is dead and you can't see her," he or she could possibly have a catastrophic reaction - thinking they are hearing this news for the first time.

At a facility in which I worked, one of the residents wanted to call her husband – about a hundred times a day (or so it seemed) – so one of the Aides on the unit dialed the number of her home and her sister answered. The sister informed the resident that her husband had died 27 years earlier. In the resident's mind, this news was the first time she had heard it. She had no memory of her husband having died 27 years earlier. For about a day she walked throughout the unit crying – telling everyone that her husband had died and the funeral was going to be the next day.

<u>Sleep Disturbance</u>. This is a common malady of the Alzheimer's patient. Oftentimes the patient is awake and up roaming throughout the night and during the day he or she wants to doze or sleep, somewhat like a baby who has days and nights mixed up. This can be very frustrating to the family or caregiver because the patient wants to sleep and not eat, or do the other things they need to do during the day. The patient can be very irritable and tired all the time. Indeed this is frustrating to

the caregiver, but here again, try to discover the cause of their not sleeping at night and the right sleep aid can almost work miracles. Trust me. I have seen this happen.

Someone may think, "Well, it is great that they are sleeping during the day, you don't have to put up with them acting up." But if they are not eating and drinking, as they should, this could be devastating. The patient can become anemic, dehydrated, and ultimately fail to thrive because they are not taking in enough nutrients to keep them alive. As a caregiver of Alzheimer's/Dementia patients, this was one of the more difficult areas of the disease I had to deal with. When the patient slept all day and was up at night it does away with any normalcy in their lives - they are not involved in activities, do not eat as well and miss times with family visits. Oftentimes, when you do awaken them during the day, they are very unstable and non-compliant. So you see, not sleeping at night causes a tremendous hardship – not only on the patient, but also on the caregiver as well.

Even though they are getting a lot of sleep, they are still exhausted because their sleep is not a restful sleep – their sleep is due to a brain disorder. The good news is that there are mild sedatives that can, in many cases, help this behavior.

<u>Sexual Inappropriateness</u>. This particular behavior can be very embarrassing for a wife or husband. In early childhood there is a period that many children go through in which they like to touch themselves. This can be very normal – it just feels good. Alzheimer's can stimulate the sensual part of the brain and patients may touch themselves inappropriately. Remember that they are losing their executive function – their ability to know what is appropriate and what is not appropriate.

I had a patient once who continually kept his hand in his pull-ups. He was 84 years of age. To anyone looking at him, this was inappropriate, but to him there was no right or wrong to it – it just felt good. It was not even a sexual thing. He was like the two-year-old who discovered that it just felt good to touch himself. The wife was embarrassed by his behavior, but to make him stop created a lot of agitation for him, so I suggested she place a blanket over him when he was up in his wheelchair, and when other people were around. I also told her that if her friends noticed him doing this, to simply tell them it is a part of his disease and it will pass; but until it does, that is just the way it is. To people that matter, they will understand.

The less attention that is brought to this behavior, the better off everyone is. I know it is very difficult for the spouse and family members when their loved one is exhibiting this behavior publicly, but this will pass.

I must say at this point, that for more alert Alzheimer's patients, they may be very verbally inappropriate. They may say words that would never have passed their lips before Alzheimer's. I have had grown children cry because they were hearing their godly mother use vulgarity as if it was nothing. This is part of the disease. When we learn what creates this behavior, we can minimize it. Remember that disagreement or arguing with them is a precursor to this type of behavior. To scold them is futile – it will only create an agitated situation. Remind them this is wrong and unacceptable - then let it go.

It is not important for you to be right. Don't argue with them! Remember that it is the disease - not your loved one.

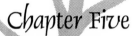

Chapter Five

Dementias That Have Alzheimer's Characteristics

Because Alzheimer's carries with it many symptoms that are similar to other types of Dementia, I want to share some of these conditions that may cause you to believe your loved one has Alzheimer's, when in fact he or she does not.

<u>Pick's Disease</u>. Dr. Arnold Pick, a German neurologist, first described this disease in 1892. While there is not the normal loss of memory with this particular type of Dementia, as in Alzheimer's, there is a loss in inhibition, impulse control and language skills.

Patients with Pick's Disease are more likely to be uninhibited, saying inappropriate things at inappropriate times. They tend to eat whatever they can get their hands on, cry a lot and are insensitive to other's feelings. One lady told me that her mother, who had been diagnosed with Pick's Disease, acted like the whole world revolved around her - no one or nothing else mattered. She also stated this was totally opposite of how her mother had been all her life – before, she had been loving, giving, always thinking of others before herself.

At the present time there are no effective drug therapies to treat Pick's Disease, but keeping patients active, physically and mentally, has been a tremendous help in controlling their impulsive behaviors.

<u>Frontal Lobe Dementia</u>. Is caused by a mutation of chromosome 17 (an abnormal tissue growth). This mutation can cause a degeneration of frontal lobe cells that can cause Dementia.

There are personality changes that occur with Frontal Lobe Disease that are not typically a part of the patient's personality. They have little regard to the feelings of others and may have expressionless faces. You may share some exciting news with them and they may not even show the slightest bit of interest in what you have shared. Or they may laugh at serious situations or sad news. They are very rigid in their thinking and can become very ritualistic in behavior, such as repeating the same action over and over or folding a towel again and again. They may be sexually promiscuous, making inappropriate gestures, saying inappropriate things to you, health care workers, or people of the opposite sex. They may steal things impulsively and if they are living in a Nursing Home or an Assisted Living Facility, they may go into another patient's room and take jewelry, food, clothes, etc.

<u>Frontal Temperal Lobe Dementia</u>. This type of Dementia can start very early, even in the 30's for some patients. This particular Dementia is often confused with Alzheimer's because there is some loss of memory from the very onset. A patient may have language problems, not be able to say correct words or finish sentences.

There may also be personality changes and loss of inhibition. They also have short-term memory loss, so you can see Frontal Temporal Lobe Dementia can be misdiagnosed as Alzheimer's. There seems to be, however, one distinguishing symptom called hypochondriosis. This is a big word meaning they constantly think they have a serious illness, such as cancer, heart disease, or symptoms that will lead to their having a stroke. This causes them to live in a continuous state of fear every day during their waking hours. The word hypochondriac is a common word that indicates a person has symptoms of every disease they hear about, but hypochondriosis zeros in on one serious disease that makes them believe they are dying. They have a multiple amount of complaints that, when checked out, are nothing serious at all. Alzheimer's drugs to assist with the disease itself are not very helpful, but anti-psychotic drugs and anti-depressants are very helpful with the psychosis.

<u>Lewy Body</u>. Another type of Dementia that has symptoms so closely related to Alzheimer's disease that it is still not certain if Lewy Body Dementia is a distinct syndrome or just a variation of Alzheimer's disease or Parkinson's disease.

Dementia with Lewy Bodies are abnormal areas of the cerebral cortex which is the snake-like ridges of the brain. It sometimes has the same characteristics as Alzheimer's disease. These wave-like ridges of the external surface of the brain, known as the cerebral cortex, is where the personality and intelligence is found; along with motor functions, planning ability and sense of touch. If this area of the brain is damaged by any means, it results in losing the ability to control body movements such as walking or using the hands. You can develop tremors where the hands shake. This type of tremor resembles Parkinson's disease.

Treatment for Lewy Body Dementia is difficult because drugs used to control the shaking caused by Parkinson's disease can lead to hallucinations and delusions; while drugs used to control the psychotic symptoms can make the involuntary movements much worse.

<u>Parkinson's Disease</u>. Rigidity, tremors, poor balance, and involuntary movements characterize this form of Dementia. Parkinson's can affect people in their 40's or younger. One of the most recent celebrities who have publicly talked about his Parkinson's is Michael J. Fox.

This disease is seldom confused with Alzheimer's, but a person who is not aware of the patient's history might confuse the Dementia that may come at the late stage of Parkinson's with Alzheimer's, if the tremors are controlled with medications. Dementia does not always come with Parkinson's.

<u>Vascular Dementia</u>. This is the most common form of Dementia that depicts some of the same characteristics as Alzheimer's. Untreated high blood pressure causes 50% of all Vascular Dementia and this Dementia is more prevalent among Afro-Americans.

Vascular Dementia can develop as a result of problems with circulation of blood in the brain due to hemorrhage, blood clots, poorly controlled diabetes, high cholesterol and high blood pressure. These problems can cause brain tissue to die as a result of a lack of oxygen that is caused by a disruption of circulation. A person's cognitive or decision-making ability is affected. The cognitive ability is the ability to make appropriate decisions.

Vascular Dementia occurs usually after a patient has had a stroke or a series of TIA's (Transient Ischemic Attacks). Initially, the patient may exhibit short-term memory loss, lethargy, or confusion, but come out of it and then appear perfectly normal within an hour. To show how quickly TIA's can occur, I had a patient who had several of these mini-strokes and by the time the EMT's arrived to transport her to the Emergency Room she was fine and refused to go to the hospital. TIA's are caused by tiny blood clots or narrowing of the arteries; or there may be an inflammatory process going on. Dizziness and confusion, along with slurred speech and lack of coordination may be the visible symptoms of a TIA, but these symptoms should go away within a few minutes or an hour. If they do not, medical help should be sought at once, as your loved one has probably had a full-fledged stroke and immediate treatment is indicated.

Multi Infarct Dementia. Is caused by small blood clots to vessels in the brain and is common in people with high blood pressure. Symptoms may include severe headaches, memory problems, getting lost, wandering, loss of bowel and bladder control, and emotional problems such as crying inappropriately, problems with money (large amounts of money may be paid for simple services).

With Multi Infarct Dementia, a diagnosis can be confirmed with a CAT Scan (X-ray) of the brain. This can aid the Physician in the early diagnosis and treatment of the disease and prevent further damage, but it must be noted that damage already done is irreparable damage.

Subdural Hematomas. This is bleeding or a large blood clot that occurs under the tough fibrous tissue that protects the brain. My father died as the result of a Subdural Hematoma. He exhibited the classic symptoms throughout the day before his death that night. He was nauseated, confused, felt the room was smoky or the television was snowy. Around

Neurosyphilis is more commonly called syphilis of the brain. This condition may be caused as the result of a lack of treatment early on. Syphilis can be cured with antibiotics, but left untreated for a long period of time may cause the treatment not to be as successful.

Still there are a few other things that can cause Dementia or confusion. Depression, alcohol abuse, urinary tract infections, traumatic injury to the head, schizophrenia, delirium, or poisoning may all cause short-term Dementia or long-term Dementia or memory loss. If the patient receives treatment, the Dementia or memory loss symptoms may disappear.

You can see that Doctors sometimes walk a tight rope in trying to diagnose the right kind of Dementia your loved one has. Some of the treatments may or may not work, but they have to keep trying with medications – somewhat a trial and error process to get your loved one the exact medication that will allow optimum quality of life. Patience on your part is oftentimes needed until the right medication is found.

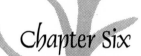

Chapter Six

Placing Your Loved One
In A Facility For Care

When a family decides to place a loved one in a Nursing Home or Assisted Living Facility, the family needs to know that just because the loved one is confused does not negate the fact that he or she still deserves to be treated with respect and dignity. He or she should be given as much independence as possible and their privacy is to be respected.

Hopefully, the knowledge you gain from this chapter will empower you to give the right kind of care and be a valuable resource if you do have to relinquish this care to professional caregivers. Your loved one deserves to continue receiving the kind of care that will afford the very best quality of life which can possibly be experienced in their last years.

Every Alzheimer's or Dementia patient has a different level of capabilities. While some are very high functioning and can follow simple directions, there are others that may not be able to do much at all.

If your loved one is admitted to a Nursing Home or Assisted Living Facility, a Registered Nurse has to do an initial assessment of the patient, because it is with this assessment that all care, medical and physical, is initiated. If there are wounds, bruises, sores, skin tears, long nails, or the patient is dirty and smelly, all this is documented so that the staff will know how the patient was when he or she arrived to the facility. This assessment is of utmost importance later on, especially if a family member notices a bruise, skin tear or wound. The staff can refer back to the initial assessment and see that it was there upon admission. If help with feeding, "toileting", or ambulating (walking) is needed, this assessment will reveal that as well.

This initial assessment will aid in helping caregivers know how much assistance a new resident in their building requires. If the patient is confused, he or she may be very resistant to care. There are steps that caregivers can do to then assist with the care of your loved one.

Above all things, the caregivers need to get to know the resident so they will know how the resident will respond to care. When I was the Director on the Haven, I had a form that was given to every Nursing Assistant when I admitted a new resident. This form contained the following information on the new resident: name, how many children he or she had, the guardian's names(s), previous employment history, hobbies, where they lived, their special abilities (such as dancing, singing or playing an instrument), how ambulatory they were, if they needed to use a walker or wheelchair, if they had skin disorders, if they could communicate, dress themselves or not. This tool was a valuable source of information for my staff to know and enabled them to give optimum care. Approach and communication were two of the more important things the staff had to develop with each new patient and these forms certainly assisted greatly in this process. Remember, these were total strangers to the staff and it was an adjustment for everyone – patient, family, and staff alike.

Whenever a person is admitted to a Nursing Home or an Assisted Living Facility, it is very important that you have confidence that the staff has been trained in knowing how to **approach** your loved one and **communicate** with him or her – verbally and non-verbally. If the staff has not had this training, your loved one may not have all their needs met. I cannot say it enough – your loved one should be placed, when you can no longer provide the adequate care needed, in a facility that has staff that has been trained to give appropriate care and in a safe way.

Approach is one of the most important aspects of caregiving for a confused resident. The patient should be approached in a calm, friendly manner. Eye contact should be made and you should always tell the patient what you are going to do. If you walk up to them and start touching them, they may get afraid and combative. Some people do not want to be touched at all and this must be respected. Talk slowly and clearly, using short, simple sentences. If your loved one does not want to do what you want them to do at this time, go do something else and come back to them later. If your loved one does not want to eat right at the designated time, put the food in the microwave and come back to it later. If you argue with them it will end up in a bad situation and your day will have had a bad beginning or a drastic, dramatic turn for the worse.

If your loved one is in a Nursing Home, he or she deserves respect, privacy and dignity. Doors should be closed when they are being showered or bathed. Curtains should be pulled while they are being dressed. You certainly would not want the landscaping people to be able to look into a resident's room and see them with no clothes on. Just because they are confused does not mean they do not deserve the same respect, privacy, and dignity as a person who is not confused.

A part of any patient maintaining dignity is by being allowed to do as much for himself or herself as possible. They may not remember how to prepare their food, but they still may be able to feed themselves. They may not be able to button buttons, but they may still be able to put on their shirt and then be assisted with the buttoning. They might not be able to tie their shoes, but they may still be able to put them on. Everything they are capable of doing, they should be allowed to do. This undoubtedly will take patience on the caregivers part because the resident might be very slow.

Patients should be asked to do things, not told they are going to do things. They should be given choices such as what they want to wear or eat. This is allowing them autonomy and independence. They should be referred to by their names, not by such terms as sweetie, honey, sugar or baby. To call them by these names is demeaning. They are adults and deserve to be treated as adults. They have lived long, productive lives, paving the way for us so that our lives are easier. Family members often use one of these terms in an enduring way – this is their loved one. But for professional care-givers to talk down to or using demeaning words or terms in reference to or in addressing them is unacceptable.

Many confused residents resist care. There are four main reasons they do this:

1. They may be fearful. The confused patient oftentimes is afraid of water – he or she may hesitate to step on a shiny floor because they perceive the floor as water or being wet. They may be afraid of the caregiver, especially if they are not approached in a kind, gentle way. They may be afraid of being hurt, especially if they have previously been physically abused.
2. The second thing the confused person may be experiencing is frustration. He or she may be frustrated that someone else has to help them or that they cannot complete tasks on their own.

3. The third thing that causes the confused patient to resist care is fatigue. He or she may be tired and not want to be bothered. If you insist, they may cry, shout at you, or become physical if you try to force them.
4. Fourthly, the patient may not be feeling well. He or she may have a urinary tract infection or may not have slept well through the night.

There may be other reasons, but these four are the most prevalent. If you can try to put yourself in their situation, how frustrated would you be if a part of you did not understand why people had to do things for you? These poor, confused people are so full of emotions that they cannot vent, except for being combative or inappropriate. They are doing the best they can with what they have.

<u>Communicating</u> with the patient with Dementia or Alzheimer's can be difficult, but it can be done. What if you were in a foreign country and you could not speak the language – you did not understand what was being said to you and you could not get people to understand you? How frustrating would that be? I have been to other countries on several occasions and I became frustrated due to the fact I could not understand what was being said to me.

Alzheimer's slowly destroys the patient's cognitive abilities such as thinking, memory, language, and understanding. We have to communicate differently to the patient with Dementia than with people who are not mentally impaired.

When we talk to the Alzheimer's patient, we must speak in slow, "short" sentences. They cannot process long sentences. Information from A to B is incomplete because of the plaque build-up on the brain cells which causes a break in the transmission of information. Thus, the patient does not understand all you are saying. You may have to repeat the sentence several times before they actually can understand. Here again, they are doing the best they can with what they have to work with. Always offer a hand and get eye level. If they are sitting, kneel down or sit in a chair opposite them. If they are not "touchy, feely" persons, don't touch them without asking. To do so may cause agitation or combativeness. Yes or no questions are good to ask. It will help them to maintain some autonomy by making a choice.

Early in the disease, the Alzheimer's patient understands 3 out of 4 words. Later in disease, 1 out of 2 words is understood.

One day I walked through the unit on the Haven and there were five women sitting on a sofa. As I walked by I said, "Good morning ladies. It is a beautiful day." I went into a nearby room and

I heard one of the ladies on the sofa ask, "What did she say?" One of the others replied, "She said 'morning.'" Someone else inserted, "She said something about day." I realized how much they had missed of what I had really said. Each time I spoke to them after that, I stopped, got down in front of them and spoke to each one so they would understand what I was saying. I had spoken <u>eight</u> words and between these five ladies, <u>two</u> words were heard.

Taking away, as much as possible, the noise surrounding patients is helpful in being able to communicate with them. Televisions, radios, or people playing loud games can be distracting and the patient cannot hear you. If the television or radio is on, ask the patient if you may turn it down.

Communication can also be done in other ways, such as non-verbally. Smiling can make the Dementia patient think you are happy, whereas a frown may make them think you are upset with them.

If you stand in front of them with your arms folded, they may interpret that as you being angry with them. Or if you talk too fast or your movements are quick, they may interpret that as you being impatient with them. This may cause the patient to be very fearful or frustrated because they don't know what is going on.

While working in an Alzheimer's unit in a western state, I received a patient from another state and she had been in a very abusive situation. She would cower and cover her face and head every time one of my staff or myself walked into the room. I can truly say I had never felt more compassion for a person in my life. I immediately had a staff meeting and shared with them how this lady was to be cared for – gently, lovingly, and patiently. If a staff member who was assigned to her was having a bad day, then that staff member was not to go into her room because my goal was for her to feel safe. All "wanderers" were not allowed to enter her room. Eventually she came out of her room and mingled with the other residents. What a happy day that was for her daughter who had rescued her from the abusive situation.

Alzheimer's patients are often childlike and will not fight back or defend themselves when they are being abused. The people in the facility from which she was transferred knew very little about Alzheimer's. They felt she was deliberately behaving in an inappropriate manner. Many people feel this way. After all, for their entire lives they have not been inappropriate. Many caregivers and family members often times believe the confused patient should be able to control inappropriateness in any form – even if the loved one has Alzheimer's.

That is why knowledge is so important. It gives us the power to understand that their actions are the result of a disease process and to react in an appropriate manner so that the patient is not hurt.

Modeling is a form of communication that can also be highly effective. In modeling, you literally show the patient what you want him or her to do. For example, if you want them to brush their teeth, you go through the motion. If you want them to comb their hair, put the brush in their hand and you guide in brushing through their hair. Showing them how will help them do many of the tasks you are trying to get them to do. Modeling also cuts down on the stress level and can curb an agitated situation when you are trying to get patients to do things for themselves.

Remember that their autonomy and independence should be encouraged for as long as possible. Also, remember that things such as buttons may be difficult for them to work with – ask them if you can help.

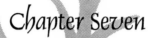

Chapter Seven

Questions To Ask When Considering Placement For Your Loved One

When you have to admit your loved one to a Long-term Care or an Assisted Living Facility, do not be timid about asking questions. It is important that you know how the facility operates and how your loved one will be cared for on a daily basis.

If a Nursing Home is not willing to answer your questions up front, that facility may not be the place for your loved one. You need to have peace of mind. If you go home at night and lay awake worrying that your mom or dad is not getting adequate care you will be in a mental, living nightmare.

The questions I have written about are valid questions. Copy them and take them with you in your search. When you find a facility that can answer your questions to your complete satisfaction, then that is probably the place for your love one to live.

What are the Nursing Assistants to patient ratio?

All Assisted Living and Long-term Care Facilities, such as Nursing Homes are in business to make a profit and they will make a profit no matter what they have to cut in services. Unfortunately, one of the first things to be cut back is staff.

The State mandates that there has to be a certain amount of Nursing Assistants for a given number of patients. Usually a ratio of "12 to 1", "10 to 1", "8 to 1", or "5 to 1". It really depends on the activity or the amount of care the patients need. If a ratio is 15 patients to 1 Nursing Assistant, and the patients are all essentially bed-bound or "total care" dependant, then there is no possible way these 15 people can get the care they need in an 8-hour shift from 1 person. As a result, they are generally divided up so that the Aide only has maybe 5 or 6 of these people and the rest of their patients are people who can somewhat help themselves.

When there is a cut back in staff, services, or even supplies, it is your family members who suffer. With fewer supplies to meet the needs of patients and fewer staff to care for them, patients are more vulnerable, more subject to falls and injury. This is why the question of staff to resident ratio is so important. When you leave the facility in which your loved one will possibly live out the rest of his or her life, you need assurance that they will be safe and cared for – you deserve peace of mind.

How is your staff trained to care for people who are confused?

This is one of the more important questions you need to ask. A staff needs special training, apart from the basic C.N.A. training, in order to effectively care for confused patients. If the person you are questioning responds, "Our staff are all trained, Certified Nursing Assistants and they are afforded monthly in-services," – they are telling you that they have had and are getting on-going training for the general care of the resident who needs assistance with his or her activities of daily living. If the person with whom you are talking does not tell you that the staff has been specially trained to redirect, communicate verbally and non-verbally, show patients dignity and respect, help patients maintain autonomy, individuality, and independence – more than likely, they have not had the specialized training which is so necessary in working with those with Alzheimer's or Dementia. **A good staff knows how to do all these things – A GREAT STAFF WILL DO THEM.**

What activities are offered?

Activities are a very important part of the Nursing Home. They stimulate the body and mind. It is of utmost importance that you place your loved one in a facility that offers a variety of activities. Many people in Nursing Homes and Assisted Living Facilities are depressed because of lack of activities. They sit and stare at each other aimlessly with a hopeless face. They often beam when someone stops and talks with them or just shows a little interest.

If you visit your loved one often and the residents are sitting around doing nothing, this is a sign that there are too few activities. The Activities

Department is not a priority in many facilities. When I worked in New Jersey, for 220 residents we had over 45 activity persons on staff. My unit of 30 Alzheimer residents had 3-4 Activity Aides during the day and if there was a call out, my staff filled in. They were trained to do this. The Corporation that owned the facility I worked in was big on activities. They knew the importance of them to the well being of the residents. Mental and physical stimulation is of utmost importance to keep your loved one as active for as long as possible. If you look at a facility that has 100 or more residents and they have 1 activity person – beware.

If you are not concerned that your loved one be stimulated and given diversion that can help him or her to be more alert and active for a longer period of time, then the activities department does not matter. But I cannot help but believe that because you do care for your loved one, activities are an important part of the entire package when you make your final decision.

Activities keep the patients moving and keeps their minds as alert as possible. This is just as important as the medication they are taking. Activities cut down on depression, anxiousness, combativeness, and general laziness. Activities can also make them move, stimulate them mentally and give them something to do on a daily basis.

I realized one day how important the Activities Department was in my building. We took the residents to a popular restaurant in a nearby town. Out of my 30 residents, 14 went on the outing. They were like different people. They were so excited and some talked much more while at the restaurant - these were some of my residents who were generally not friendly at all. I was amazed. So I say "Hurray for activities!"

Is there a dietician on staff?

As people age they often do not eat well – their sense of sight and smell can be impaired, thus food is not as tasty or does not have a pleasurable smell. They often do not drink fluids, as they should. Dehydration is a common diagnosis when older adults have to make a visit to the emergency room.

If patients in Nursing Homes and Assisted Living Facilities are not offered fluid, they can go all day with only a few ounces of fluid. This is a travesty, because they simply are not offered water or a juice. In most cases, they would drink if it was available; but if they are confused and wheel chair bound, they may not be able to get their own water and often they cannot ask for it either. Here again, staffing is so important. If there is adequate staffing and adequate training, residents will receive better care.

Every CNA and Nurse should be able to recognize the signs of dehydration and alert someone so that the patient can receive help. If you lift up some skin on the forearm and it relaxes slowly and the patient's skin is extremely dry, this is a sign of dehydration. So is excessive, foul smelling, condensed urine. These are indicators of things we as caregivers can see and smell. If staff is properly trained, they will be cognizant of these things and alert the Nurse or Doctor, and the patient can receive the needed care.

A dietician can actually write orders for routine increases of fluids, high protein and high calorie drinks; and Doctors have no problem signing off on these. A dietician can also order blood work that will reveal dehydration or protein levels (these orders are carried out only with the Doctor's approval). If there is a low protein level, powders with extra protein can be put in the patient's fluids and this will aid in the healing of wounds.

So you can see that a dietitian is a very important person for a Nursing Home Staff.

What is your survey record?

This should be available for you to read and is usually in the lobby in plain sight. Each year, a team of Nurses that work for the State come into every facility (Long-term Care and Assisted Living), and make sure the Facilities are meeting all the requirements. These requirements include such areas as: proper documentation, proper medical care, proper staffing, proper record keeping, proper diets, proper wound care, proper cleanliness, proper food temperatures, proper maintenance, etc.

If there are things found wrong, the facility can be given deficiencies. These deficiencies range from minor to major, with the more major ones carrying monetary fines that are imposed until the facility can make acceptable corrections. The worst event that can happen in a facility is what is called a "sentinel event." This is where gross negligence is involved, such as a patient getting out and wandering away from the facility and freezing to death. This is a "sentinel event."

You can ask to see a survey record and the latest one is usually visible when you walk into the building. You can ask for the last 3 years. You might see a pattern of neglect, abuse, or poor maintenance. Remember that this is where your loved one is going to live and make his or her home. How would you want your loved one's home taken care of? How would you care for your loved one? At the very least, you should expect your loved one to receive appropriate medical care to keep him or her at optimum health and that this care be administered with respect and dignity. Take a note pad and write down what you see and what you are told. Go home and write down questions. Then go back and ask these questions. Above all, you want your loved one in a safe, caring, and clean environment.

Will there be a Doctor on staff to notify in case of emergencies? Will he or she meet with family at their request if the family has questions?

Every patient admitted to a Nursing Home or Assisted Living Care Facility has to have a personal Physician. Nursing Homes have a Medical Director who may or may not see patients in the facility. Most patients see their Doctor monthly, some every other month, and some on an as-need-to-see basis.

These Doctors come in and if there are problems, they are often not addressed while the Doctor is there because he or she comes in and may visit 20 people in a very short period of time. The Doctor can be in-and-out without the Nursing staff even being aware that he or she has been in the building, especially if the Doctor comes early in the morning while the Nursing staff is passing medications or doing blood sugar checks.

You, as a family member can actually know when the Doctor is going to make rounds and be there to discuss your loved one's condition. This will take planning, but you are entitled to know what is going on with your loved one. Just because you have entrusted your loved one to the care of a facility and its staff does not relinquish your rights as a family member to be an intricate part of their care.

Family members can choose to take the loved one to a Doctor outside the Nursing Home or Assisted Living Facility. The family can also choose to use any Doctor who comes to the facility to see their loved one, if the Doctor is willing to add them to his or her services.

Apart from the Medical Director, there are usually 2-3 Physicians who offer their services to the Nursing Home or Assisted Living Facility. These Doctors generally come in every 1-3 months to see patients and write new orders. They will also come if the staff feels a patient needs to be seen.

The downside to this is that the Doctors come in to see the patients, ask them questions, and the patients generally answer, "I'm okay," "I don't have any complaints," or "I feel fine." The Nursing staff is usually so busy that they are not a part of this interaction. But if your loved one is admitted to the Nursing Home under the care of one of these Doctors, then the Nurses can call their offices or any other time for any problem that may arise. I felt it was important that my residents have a Doctor that would come to my building because it is not always convenient to take the patient out.

Is there a Podiatrist that comes to the facility?

Podiatrists are usually called on as needed, but in some facilities they do come in every six weeks or so, to keep the patients' toenails clipped.

It is important for families to ask that a Podiatrist see their loved one. If residents are extremely confused, they may have no way of informing anyone how much pain they may be in if they have an ingrown toenail, long toenails that are curling under, bunions, or corns. Being seen on a routine basis can prevent a lot of suffering for the patient.

It must be noted here that if your loved one has diabetes, the staff should not be clipping toenails due to the possibility of cutting the skin and the resident getting an infection.

What is the process when my loved one can no longer remain in an Assisted Living or Nursing Home Facility?

When a patient has to be moved, a 30-day notice (in writing) has to be given. The only exception would be if the resident had to be sent to a Mental Health facility. This is equivalent to their being sent out to the hospital. The family is notified that this is occurring. This is discussed in more detail later in this chapter.

Is there a history of abuse by staff to patients?

We would like to believe this does not take place in Nursing Homes and Assisted Living Facilities, but unfortunately it does. Even with all the monitoring that has been put in place by various

States, Corporations that run the facilities, and the Nursing Homes and Assisted Living Facilities themselves, there is still negligence and abuse of all kinds – physical, mental, and emotional.

One evening when I was a Supervisor on the Advanced Alzheimer's unit in a Nursing Home, I walked by a room and heard a "slap." The patient began to cry and mumbled, "Don't hurt me." I immediately knew the Nursing Assistant had hit her. I went into the room and told the Nursing Assistant to leave the building. She looked at me and said, "She has Alzheimer's. She doesn't even remember what happened." I responded, "She might not, but I will, so leave the building." I worked as a Nursing Assistant the remainder of the shift in order to cover her patient load.

This is one example of gross abuse, but there are also other kinds of neglect and abuse that takes place. Some of the areas include: dirty toe nails that are long and ingrown, dirty finger nails, hair not combed, clothes not cleaned and patients wearing the same clothes day after day, patients allowed to have smelly body odor, encrusted feces on them and under their nails, encrusted food around their mouths, ear wax, eyes having dry matter in them, dirty bandages on wounds, skin tears unexplained, falls unexplained, dehydration, inactivity, putting incontinent briefs (diapers) on continent patients so staff won't have to get them up during the night to take them to bathroom, giving preferential treatment to some patients (some family members will actually pay Nursing Assistants to give their family members special treatment – this is under the table and most Administrators do not know this is going on), discrimination and reverse discrimination (as a RN who has worked in 5 Nursing Homes, I have witnessed both).

How is this stopped? *Education, education, education, and observation, observation, observation.* If you place a confused, demented loved one in a facility and don't visit to see how he or she is treated and cared for, they are at the mercy of the staff of that Nursing Home or Assisted Living Facility. These caregivers are not emotionally attached to your loved one, so when patients get difficult to handle, staff may abuse them.

There is a phenomenal amount of CNA turnover in Nursing Homes. Agency Nursing Assistants are used all too often, so total strangers are caring for your loved ones, especially on the night shifts and weekends.

If your loved one has short-term memory loss and he or she is physically abused, they will not be able to tell anyone because they will not remember. I think of Alzheimer's like someone who is paralyzed and has no feelings in the legs. If he or she is burned or scraped, they do not know it until they see the blister or blood. They may not be able to know when, where, or how it happed. It is the same with Alzheimer's patients. They do not know and cannot tell anyone how the bruise got on their arm, leg or face. In-house investigations may not turn up very much.

If a loved one keeps coming up with bruises, skin tears or wounds – BEWARE. This is a sign that they could very well be being treated roughly, if not being abused or neglected.

Even though a patient is confused and has lost a lot of his or her short-term memory, if your loved one keeps telling you that "she hurts me," or "please help me," – LISTEN to them. If they get anxious or fearful when a caregiver comes near – check into it. They do have periods where they are cognizant or alert. They may feel things are not right, but not be able to tell you. Remember that they are communicating the best they can with a limited amount of brainpower and memory. Often they read body language more than understanding words. If a CNA who is caring for them is angry or being rough, they may feel they have caused the anger and become very afraid of the caregiver. When you visit, watch how your loved one interacts with the caregivers. This can be a good indicator of how they are being treated when you are not there.

Will we know of any and all medication changes made by the M.D.?

This is your right to ask.

Will we be called if there is a fall, whether there is physical harm or not?

This is generally policy and procedure.

Are there extra charges for supplies and if so, what is the cost of supplies that the facility provides? If my loved one is in an Assisted Living Facility and his or her personal supplies run out, what will be the cost for the facility to supply these needs?

If your loved one is wearing incontinent briefs or the Doctor has ordered Ensure three or four times a day, an Assisted Living Facility may allow you to bring these things in. The staff will use them for your family member only if they are "private pay" (Medicaid pays for this if they are not "private pay"). If these things run out, the facility will provide these things, but you will pay $1.00 - $4.00 for each incontinent brief that is used, or $3.00 - $4.00 for each serving of Ensure if it has been ordered by the Doctor. You need to remember that this is not per can, but per serving. If a can is opened, but the Doctor has ordered only 4 ounces with each meal, you will pay $6.00 - $12.00 for a full can to be used over the course of the day for your loved one. You are paying for convenience and administration.

In some Assisted Living Facilities there is a charge, per day, for administration of routine medication. In one facility where I worked, if the patient was on 5 or more drugs, it was $5.00 per day. It was more with more drugs. Some of my residents could pay up to $300.00 per month just to be given their medications on a daily basis.

All the things you were doing routinely for your loved one at home now has a price. Not all facilities charge the same, so you need to look into as many facilities as possible when you have to put your family member in a Long-term Care or Assisted Living Facility. If they are accepted on Medicaid, these charges do not apply.

Ask for a list of ALL charges that can or may be incurred while your loved one is in the facility, since it could eventually run into a great deal of money.

How many days notice will I receive if my loved one has to be moved?

How many days notice will I receive if my loved one's disease process becomes such that they are a danger to themselves or someone else and they must be moved? If this happens, will you help me find placement for them? If my loved one has to be moved, how long will I have to find another facility? Can my loved one stay here when he or she has to go on Medicaid?

In all facilities, a minimum of a 30-day notice has to be given in writing to family members when their loved one has advanced with his or her Dementia to the point that they must be moved. Most facilities that are genuinely caring, will at least give you names of places that you might contact that can care for your loved one. Usually a facility that makes a recommendation about another facility for your loved one knows a lot about that facility and you can trust the recommendation. If your loved one no longer has funds, it may be a bit more difficult to find placement for them because most Nursing Homes have a percentage of Medicaid they can take, and if they have met their quota, they may not be able to accept your loved one. If you find a Nursing Home you like, be persistent. A lot of things change on a weekly basis in Long-term Care Facilities. Even if there is a room change within the facility you must be notified (sometimes there has to be a room change due to personal differences or personality differences – some people just cannot live together).

Once you have been notified by the facility that your loved one has to be moved, begin searching ASAP for a new facility. Get the name of your loved one on lists. You can call the Department of Health and Human Services in your State and they can help.

Probably the three main reasons you would have to move your loved one are: 1) change in health status; 2) change in finances (going to Medicaid from private pay; or 3) change in mental status that would cause him or her to be dangerous to self or others.

Will there be repercussions if I complain about care being given my loved one?

Many family members are afraid to complain to Administration. For example, there is a woman who lives close to me and her mother is in a Nursing Home in a nearby town. She visited her mother a few days ago and her mother's roommate had finger-painted with feces on the walls, furniture, and even on this lady's mother's clothes in the dresser drawers. The daughter called her sister who has guardianship of the mother and shared what she had found when she entered their mother's room. My neighbor wanted to complain to the Administrator simply because the feces was not fresh but dried, so she knew it had been there for a while. However her sister, the guardian, told her not to complain and reminded her that their mother was on Medicaid, she was not a "private pay," so for her not to complain. These women are afraid that if they complain they will have to move their mother, who also has Alzheimer's, or possibly have to take her home. They fear their loved one will get the repercussions from the staff if they complain. This is a fear of many family members who have loved ones in Nursing Home Facilities.

I have a friend whose mother had Alzheimer's and was in an Assisted Living Facility for 2 ½ years. The mother declined in health and my friend had to move her mother from the Assisted Living Unit to a Nursing Home. Within months, her mother had declined drastically and became totally wheel chair bound. As a result of a fall and bruises the staff could not explain, the patient was sent to the hospital, where she died within a short period of time. When my friend complained, the staff of the Nursing Home brushed her off as being a difficult daughter. This happens all too often.

If you have a "gut feeling" that things are not as they should be – whatever fears you have – go to someone with your concern. What people don't know they cannot fix. If the things you find that are wrong continue, call the State. This is your right, and ultimately you may save your loved one's life. Just because people are confused, difficult to care for, or are in need of total care, does not predispose them to abuse by you as a family member or a caregiver in a facility. These people have lived their lives and have overcome many adversities – they deserve respect, dignity, patience, and kindness from their caregivers.

Do you have a Hospice that comes to your building?

When your loved one reaches the very end stage of the Alzheimer's disease, Hospice may need to be called in to assist the facility and family during these final hours. Most Nursing Homes and Assisted Living Facilities have a contract with a Hospice organization, but you have the right to use any Hospice that you wish. You may have to take your loved one home if you choose a Hospice that is not contracted with the facility. Another thing to consider here: if your loved one has lived in the facility for a while, that may be home to him or her. It may be easier for family to allow them to die in their room, than take them home.

Hospice is a wonderful organization that can make sure your loved one is not suffering, and that you as a family member can be guided through the dying process with understanding and peace. This also takes a lot of the strain off the Nursing Home staff. Your loved one will get all the extra care that is needed at this time by trained professionals who deal with terminal illness on a daily basis.

Hospice will also allow you the time to get everything in order to make the transition from life to death as easy as possible for the loved one, you and other family members.

Who will be privy to information in relation to my loved one?

X

The last issue I want to discuss in relation to your loved one being placed in a Health Care Facility and the question which should be asked and answered before making such a decision is the Privacy Issue.

NO information is to be given out in regard to your loved one without a consent form having been signed. This protection has been brought about by the "Right To Privacy Act."

The staff is not to speak of your loved one in relation to their care or behavior in front of anyone else except to you or another Health Care professional who might need to know something to help give more enhanced care.

Some family members will argue with Nursing staff about information they want, but cannot get because they do not have guardianship or are not the legal power of attorney. Nursing Homes, Assisted Livings and Hospitals CANNOT give any information in regard to the patients in their care – even to some family members.

I feel stories help people to understand a concept, so I will share one to illustrate.

When I was nursing in a hospital in a western state, two Nurses got on an elevator where there was a woman and gentleman already on. As the door closed, one of the Nurses stated, "I could not believe how that patient in ICU bled out this morning. The Doctor said his heart exploded."

The woman on the elevator got off and went to the ICU unit, not knowing that it was her husband the Nurses were discussing. When she found out, she was devastated. She was also angered that the two Nurses had discussed her husband's death on the elevator. It was mumbled throughout the Hospital that a man's heart had exploded in ICU.

The wife sued the Hospital and won a large sum of money. The two Nurses lost their jobs.

If you want to engage in an argument with Nursing staff – trying to get information about loved ones – you are fighting a losing battle. Medical professionals have been trained and retrained to maintain the patient's privacy and the bottom line is that you would not want your loved one in a place that didn't.

The guardian and power of attorney are the only ones to whom information can be released, except other family members whose names have been put on a list that allows them to receive such information from the staff.

If you desire information about a loved one in a facility, contact the family member who is privy to the information. Family members can freely share information among themselves, but the caregiver cannot.

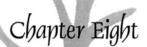

Chapter Eight

Stories Of Patients With Dementia

In this chapter, I will be sharing with you some stories of people for whom I have had the privilege of caring.

These stories of people with Alzheimer's and Dementia are shared with the hope that you will see that some of the behaviors exhibited by your loved one are not unique to them. There are other family members that have walked the road before you with different behaviors such as combativeness, anger, agitation, paranoia, inappropriate language, etc.

People with Alzheimer's or Dementia are often very volatile – they are often unpredictable – they often do not know moment from moment how they are going to act or react to a given situation, and neither does the caregiver. The more which is learned, the more prepared you will be to deal with these situations and stories are an excellent way to convey concepts and principles. The stories in this chapter will assist you in seeing how quickly a patient may become difficult to deal with or how he or she can become dangerous to those around them and some of the challenges caregivers face. Every phase of Dementia or Alzheimer's carries with it challenges and education is so very important to know how to deal with these challenges. Stories are an excellent method of education.

In the Earlier Stage, attitudes and temperaments can be different. In the Middle Stage, behavior can be the challenge. In the Late Stage, the physical care can be the challenge. And the End Stage can emotionally wear on a family with tremendous strain. So these are various challenges that have to be dealt with from the beginning to the end of the disease process.

Another desire I have in sharing these stories is to convey, to you the reader, that confused people are often vibrant, intelligent, and have often lived sacrificial lives for their children and others. As a result, the very least they deserve at this time of their lives is caring people who want to keep them safe and give to them the dignity, respect, and protection they deserve.

The Beloved

Norma came to the Assisted Living Facility as a result of her husband not being able to handle her any longer in their home setting. She was suspicious of him and accused him of things. She became extremely unpredictable and was getting out of hand. Norma was paranoid.

I went to Norma's home to conduct an assessment and knew right away that she had a lot of problems. She could not complete even one half of the mini-mental exam. She constantly got off the subject and could not follow a train of thought to complete sentences. She was struggling so very hard to be "normal." She wanted to answer the questions, but had a great deal of difficulty. After the initial assessment, Norma's husband and I decided to try Norma at the Memory Impaired Assisted Living.

The first few months were difficult. Norma wanted to go home. She tried to open all the doors, but then she began to adjust to her new home. At this time the paranoia began to worsen. She accused her husband of spending all their money, taking her money from her, seeing other women, having affairs with my staff and myself, but through all of this her husband remained very devoted. He came to see her every Monday, Wednesday and Friday. Each special occasion he sent flowers and brought her gifts, and took her to Atlantic City to gamble, which was a passion of hers. He saw that she had everything she needed and constantly reminded me that "money is not a problem, just see that she gets whatever she needs." Norma was confused, incontinent, and could get inappropriate at a moment's notice, but these things did not stop her husband from being committed to her in every way.

We all learned to love Norma, and most of the time she was a lot of fun to be around. She was truly the life of the party. The one thing that impressed me most about Norma was that she never lost her sense of humor. She never lost that twinkle in her eyes that made her uniquely Norma. Her basic temperament remained in tact until she became physically ill. She was mischievous and cute.

Though her body gave up, she fought to the end just to be Norma – the Norma who could say something that would make you laugh until it hurt – The Norma who could dance when the music came on – The Norma who had that twinkle of "mischievousness" in her eyes – The Norma who was so gentle-natured that when she was angry she would say to my staff, "Please don't let me hurt you" – The Norma who loved her husband with all her heart and when her memories of most everyone else was gone she still wanted to be with him.

This is the Norma we cared for, grew close to and watched as the disease took a little more of her away each day – The Norma we loved and eventually lost. What a privilege to have cared for such a wonderful human being. My staff and I were all better people because we knew Norma.

Finding Pennies

John was a mentally challenged gentleman who, in his later years, developed mild Dementia. He had been slow all of his life, but with aging, his condition had worsened. He was a quiet man who loved to sit in a rocking chair and watch the goings on around him. He did not participate in much, but when he was awake he really enjoyed walking.

Before John was admitted to a facility where I worked, he had a position in a convenience store, stocking the shelves. He was so proud of his job and talked about all the things he put on the shelves and the various people who patronized the store. He was proud that he had been able to make a contribution.

One day, in a conversation with one of my staff, John revealed how when he walked home from work he would try to find money that had been dropped on the ground by school children and others. This gave us an idea.

The staff, being as special as they were, started walking and sometimes driving around our building - tossing out pennies on the ground. They then would take John for walks and let him find the pennies. He would get so excited at finding those pennies. When he would find one, you would have thought he had found a piece of gold. This activity gave him purpose and it was exciting for all of us to see how John reacted when he found a penny. Finding a penny probably would not mean a lot to you or me, but to John it was definitely a "life's extra." He found a joy in this small act that most people could not understand.

By the end of the summer, he had collected a pint jar full of pennies. He, along with my staff, rolled them and he went to the store and bought some colas.

Here again, I must say that having a staff that is really in tune to the patients is invaluable. Many hours were spent with John as he walked outside and got some much-needed exercise.

Finding out what a resident or loved one truly enjoyed in the past can add many quality hours to his or her present.

The Compensating Wife

I cared for a gentleman who could not read or write. There are many people in their 70's and 80's who never finished school so this is not that uncommon. Many of them lived through the Great Depression and had to go to work to help the family or they were in World War II.

What set this gentleman apart was that all the years he could not read or write - his children were never aware of it. They, in fact, had graduated from high school and gone to prestigious universities and both were professors – but had no knowledge of their dad's inability to read or write.

You might question how could this be? But he had a wife that would read the paper to him and she handled all the finances, so the children had never seen their dad write or never heard him read. His wife compensated for him and she made him look pretty normal in this respect. When the children visited, he could carry on a knowledgeable conversation because of how his wife had read to him.

When this gentleman developed Alzheimer's, he progressed rapidly to the middle stage. His wife came to me for help and he was accepted to be a resident on the unit where I was the Wellness Nurse. On one occasion he became so disoriented and hallucinogenic that he grabbed a butter knife and another resident's cane and started screaming at us – telling us we would not take him alive. He thought we were Japanese soldiers trying to capture him. It took five men - strong men - to subdue this gentleman.

When a confused person gets combative, you really have to stay out of harm's way, especially with men. They are confused but can become very strong. They have rushes of adrenaline during this time that can make them very strong and dangerous to anyone close by or even to themselves. This rush of adrenaline often causes a "fight or flight syndrome", where the patient will fight or run. This is simply a built-in protective mechanism that we all have when we find ourselves in threatening situations.

Unfortunately, I had to have the family move this gentleman from the unit I worked on. There were other residents to be considered – residents who were very fragile and could have been severely hurt if he had been allowed to stay.

Here again, family members must understand that if their loved one becomes combative and cannot be redirected, he or she may have to be moved to a place where they will be more closely monitored. It is not because a Director or Nursing Home Administrator does not like him or her, but all residents have to be kept safe and sometimes one has to be moved for the good of the whole.

The Incessant Wanderer

I had worked in another Nursing Home before going to the Haven and I cared for a gentleman who was in the early stage of Alzheimer's. He was active, not only physically, but mentally as well.

Most of our days were spent trying to keep this gentleman out of other residents' rooms and their things. He was a lot of work to care for, but he would accept redirection well – at least for the moment, and then he was back in another patient's room. Our little ritual would then start all over again.

He enjoyed conversation and would talk to anyone who would listen. Although we could not always understand what he was saying, it was fun to talk with him.

Fortunately, his family would come in often and help us with redirecting him. One day I was in the room as his wife and daughter were looking at his memory album. What a handsome young man he had been. I told his wife I knew why she was attracted to him. He was so handsome. He glanced at me and winked.

As we looked at the pictures I noticed a "purple heart medal" on his uniform. He had been in the military during World War II and had been severely wounded. As a result he walked with a limp. As we talked about the individual photographs and we turned to the one with the "purple heart" he began to cry. His wife consoled him and we moved on. She later related to me that her husband had played a great role in breaking the German Code. My heart was touched to know I was being allowed to care for a person who had possibly saved thousands of lives in a time of war.

This is why a historical profile should be done on every resident and placed in his or her chart – so staff will know whom they are taking care of. From that day on I felt honored to care for a gentleman that had had a part in purchasing my freedom. It was on that day that I knew my staff had to know the various contributions the residents had made in their lifetime.

I did a historical profile on each resident. When I did this, it was amazing how my staff's attitude changed in relation to the care they gave the residents.

The Mother Who Felt Abandoned

Beth was in a Nursing Home in a small town. When I was asked to assess her for an Assisted Living Facility I worked in, I found her to be a very pleasant, sweet, motherly woman – calm and co-operative. She could not answer many questions on the mini-mental exam, but was ambulatory, continent, and could follow simple commands. I genuinely felt that Beth would thrive on the unit so I accepted her and she moved in with the help of her daughter and son-in-law at her side.

Everything was OK until the next day when Beth screamed at one of the Aides and cursed her, calling her the n----- word. I was shocked and when I went to her and tried to tell her how inappropriate she was, she could not believe I had confronted her with the fact of her cursing. She assured me that she would never curse. Cursing and calling someone by an inappropriate name was not something she did – even as a child. Her mother would have whipped her with a belt since that was not allowed in her home. In a matter of a few minutes she had forgotten the whole episode.

As the days passed, Beth was getting more difficult to get out of the bed. She would fight the staff, curse them and scream. She refused breakfast and normally that was not a problem, but Beth was diabetic and she had to eat breakfast.

Almost every day the staff would go through the same routine with her - this poor, frightened woman physically and verbally abused them.

After the first year, Beth had a hard time staying in the bed at night so one of the staff would sit by the bed with her until she fell asleep.

One Monday, Beth's daughter had returned from an out-of-state trip. Instead of greeting the daughter with open arms, Beth screamed and shouted profanities at her daughter, accusing her of not loving her and leaving her alone. The daughter went around the corner and wept as her mother screamed uncontrollably at the daughter she could not see.

The next day I shared this incident with the Doctor who was the Alzheimer's and Dementia Specialist. He told me Beth had felt abandoned by her daughter and all the feelings of anger she exhibited were from her believing her daughter had abandoned her. I began, with the insight gained from the Doctor, to understand Beth much better and developed a real compassion for her as a patient with Alzheimer's.

The daughter could not get over how her mother used profanity. She told me she had never heard her mother curse before Alzheimer's. She asked me why her mother was using profanity so much.

I shared with her that her mom was loosing her executive functions (the ability to control her temper, moods, and words) – the part of the brain that gave her control had been severely damaged and she could not help it. I told her that her mother was child-like in that she was like the little girl up front in church for the children's story – she is twirling around and has her dress up. The parents are devastated because her underwear is exposed. They try to get her attention and tell her to put her dress down, but she continues to twirl from side to side, not seeing one thing wrong with this behavior. Beth, I shared with her daughter, was like the little girl. There was no right or wrong to her actions. She just did it. She quickly forgets her inappropriateness and goes on as if absolutely nothing is wrong.

I told the daughter that she should really try to separate the disease from her mother and enjoy the good times she has with her – realizing that the bad times are the disease process that has taken away her mother. The daughter began to accept that she was only going to have moments in time with her mom from that moment onward.

If a person has a bad heart, we don't yell at that heart and tell it to beat correctly - to quit acting up and beat like it is supposed to. The same goes for a person with Alzheimer's. We should not yell at them and try to get them to do the right thing.

They are not capable of thinking and responding normally. Why would we treat a sick brain any differently than the person with a sick heart?

The brain is sick and not functioning, as it should. We need to have the same level of concern for the Alzheimer's patient as we do for the heart patient. Our main priority is to keep patients with Alzheimer's safe, making sure they are cared for and treated with dignity and respect.

The Sundowner

Elizabeth was a small woman and walked about the unit carrying her purse on her arm and speaking to everyone. She was very pleasant and participated in most activities. She was a dancer and enjoyed just watching other people, especially the staff when they got animated with dancing and singing.

Elizabeth was the ideal patient until about 3 or 4 o'clock in the afternoon. At that time she started "sundowning." She also would cry and beg us to let her go home. She told us that her father was going to punish her if she did not go home. In Elizabeth's mind it was 10 or 11 o'clock at night and if she did not get home she would be grounded and not allowed to go out with her friends.

With Alzheimer's patients, their memory is usually captured between the ages of 12-24 years of age. This is the period of "firsts" - first home, marriage, first child, first job, first car, first time leaving home. These were significant times in their lives so it is not unusual for them to recall their early home life when they were children or in their teenage years.

Redirection becomes a priority at this time of day. We turned on lights, closed blinds, put on big

over

band music, and started dancing. This became a daily ritual with Elizabeth.

It must be mentioned, here again, that as a general rule, when a person with Alzheimer's or Dementia is constantly desiring to go home, it is often not the home they are in or the home from which they have come to a facility, but their childhood home.

Pictures of her siblings, mother and father were so very helpful with Elizabeth. She would tell us about them everyday – to her it was like the first time she had shared this information.

Diversion and redirection were the two keys to move Elizabeth from an anxious, fearful, stressful situation to a more relaxed and happy time in her life. After a while her "sundowning" was over and she was back to normal (for her).

"Where's My Hat?"

Bud was a gentle, quiet man who constantly asked where his hat was located. It was always on his head and each time he would be so surprised when he was told that the hat was there. He was aphasic (could not express himself or finish sentences) and was extremely confused. His short-term memory was gone. Generally, he was very docile, gentle and sweet; but as he progressed in his Alzheimer's disease, he became very impatient.

As I came on the unit one morning I heard all the residents hitting the tables with silverware, chanting, "We want food, we want food." I could not believe my ears. Never had they done that before.

After getting them calmed down, table by table, I asked one of my staff what started this, and she told me Bud had started this mini riot about breakfast being late. I thought, "How could this quiet, unassuming man cause such an uproar on my unit?" This is an example of how behavior can change - and it can change quickly.

From that time I knew Bud was capable of being inappropriate if things were not done as he thought they should be done.

Bud eventually transitioned to a completely quiet world where he gave no verbal response at all. He essentially stayed a very sweet, docile gentleman until his death in 2004.

Navigation By The Stars

I cared for another resident who was highly educated and had taught "navigation by the stars" at a Naval Academy in New York. He was a very interesting and alert man, but could become extremely inappropriate if another resident got into his space. He was constantly losing things and accusing other people of taking them.

There were times he would strike at some of the residents with his cane, so I talked with the Doctor and he ordered a walker for this gentleman so the cane could be removed from his room.

If you were to sit and talk with this man, you would have no idea he had Dementia; however, the more time spent with him, the easier it was to know that he did indeed have Dementia. He would tell you about his journeys when he was young, show you pictures of boats he had built, and amaze you with his knowledge of the stars; but if he did not want you in his space, and you got in it, you were in a very dangerous place.

This gentleman would talk about other residents and make derogatory remarks to them and about them. He thought everyone else was "crazy" – but he was perfectly sane. He felt he was the most important person on the unit – it truly was all about him.

He complained so much about the care he received that I suggested to his power of attorney that he be moved to a regular Assisted Living Facility that offered help with "Activities of Daily Living." There he would have a little more freedom than he was allowed on the unit he was on. The POA agreed with me and he moved. Within two weeks he had his POA to come back to me and ask if he could move back. However, since I had given his room to a new resident and had no other vacancies, he could not come back.

If you recall, in a previous chapter that deals with the various types of Dementia, there was one that causes people to not give very much thought to what they say – they say hurtful things and do not have remorse – it truly becomes ALL about them. There are few things, according to their perception, that people who are caring for them do right. Finding fault and complaining is their daily past time. These people believe there is always something better – better care, better food, better caregivers; and when they go to what they believe is better, they sometimes realize it is not necessarily as they thought. Thus all their complaints and faultfinding start over.

"Am I Losing My Mind?"

Daniel was a friendly, outgoing man with a great personality. He loved to dance to and sing Big Band songs from the past.

When I assessed Daniel for the unit of which I was Director, he was very bright and quick at most of the answers on the mini-mental exam, but his short-term memory had definitely depreciated and he could no longer remember the last President before George Bush. He did remember, however, that the last President before Bush had been in trouble, but could not recall what kind of trouble.

Daniel's wife was already a resident of the unit and she was quite advanced with her Alzheimer's, but Daniel had been diagnosed with early stage Dementia, so he qualified to be placed on the "memory impaired early Alzheimer/early Dementia unit."

The first few months were challenging to my staff, as Daniel did not want us to do anything for his wife. He would not allow us to shower her. He got up early to go to her room to get her up and assist her dressing for each day. This, however, became a problem since she was not capable of self-care and Daniel did not give the kind of personal care to his wife that she needed.

The family was called in to assist us in knowing how to deal with this. Daniel had a son he highly respected and to whom he would listen. This son talked with his dad and told him the staff would get his mother up each day and bring her to Daniel - dressed and ready for the day. Daniel agreed to this.

As the months went by, Daniel became more and more social. He danced with the ladies on the unit, doing various dances he had done when he and they were young. Daniel even taught my staff the Fox Trot, Waltz, and the Charleston. They, in turn, tried to teach him some of the newer moves young people engage in.

One day Daniel saw me doing some charting and he came over to my table and asked if he could talk with me. I told him, certainly. He said, "Rebecca, you have never been anything but honest with me and I really need for you to be honest with me now." I assured him I would, and he asked me a question that had really been bothering him. He looked tearfully into my eyes, laid his hand on mine and asked, "Am I losing my mind?"

I looked at this man who knew in his heart that he was losing his ability to recall a lot of things and he was frightened.

I said, "No, Daniel. You are not losing your mind. You are losing some of your good memory, but so am I. I cannot recall things like I could when

I was younger, and you are older than I am, so it stands to reason you are losing a little more of your good memory than I am. No, Daniel, you are not losing your mind."

He leaned over, kissed my hand, and thanked me for relieving him of that fear.

It is very important how we answer questions. I could have told Daniel, "You know Daniel, we are all losing our minds." A flippant response like that could have sent him into a period of extreme fear and depression.

The Man Who Could Not Stay

Gene was a 62-year-old gentleman who lived at home with a caregiver, but was becoming very difficult to handle. When I arrived at his home to assess him, he was quiet, but responsive and polite. The thing that impressed me the most was that he was a gentleman in every way.

On the mini-mental exam Gene did not do well, only answering a few questions correctly. He was a man who had worked for the State, had a college education and had made a very good living for himself and his family. I felt he was a good candidate for the Assisted Living unit so his family moved him in a few days after my visit.

However, Gene did not fare well at all. The first day he became agitated and could not be redirected. In anger he pushed a resident's chair and I had to intervene. This was a minor occurrence in relation to what lay ahead. The staff was alerted to watch Gene very closely and they did.

Gene was a "wanderer." He wandered in and out of resident's rooms. He picked up things, claiming them as his, and this disturbed the residents. Although everyone on my unit was diagnosed with Alzheimer's, they were at different First and Second Stages of the disease; and some were very alert most of the time. When Gene walked into the room, the resident would begin screaming at him and that would cause Gene to become very angry and sometimes combative, wanting to fight.

Gene's behavior went on for about two months. He was not hurt and he had hurt no one, but one day he grabbed one of my Assistants. While she was trying to redirect him, he bruised her arm. He was combative and so I knew Gene could no longer remain on the unit. He was sent out to a Mental Hospital for medication adjustment. I could not accept Gene back because he was too dangerous.

Often families don't understand why their loved ones are not allowed to stay in Assisted Living situations, because the majority of the time, Assisted Living Facilities are much more attractive than are Nursing Homes or Long-term Care Facilities. However, patient safety has to be of utmost importance and therefore when a patient becomes a danger to himself, herself, or to others, then the patient must be placed in an environment which has more staff and guidelines.

Gene advanced rapidly with his Alzheimer's, and ultimately mentally weakened to the point that he could not function in any capacity.

I share this story in order to say that Alzheimer's can affect people differently, in different ways. It advances more rapidly in some than others. It is a horrible disease that takes our loved ones a little at a time until there is just a shell that they live in.

My heart went out to Gene and his family because his children were young – only in their 30's and 40's.

The Love Of A Mother

The last story I want to share with you is about a lady named Lucille. Everyone called her Ms. Lucille. She was a black lady, about 5'9" tall and had taught Nursing in a university in Georgia. Ms. Lucille was confused and forgetful, but had great memories of when her children were small and of her early years – especially during the Great Depression and World War II.

In a conversation with me she related that she had four children. When her fourth child was born her husband left one morning for work and never came home. After a few weeks she knew she was alone – left with four small children. She said at first she cried and prayed a lot, but then began to realize that in order for she and her children to survive she had to find work.

She went to the more upscale neighborhoods and offered to clean houses, empty garbage from trash cans, and sweep yards. Sometimes she was paid a nickel or a dime, and one time she swept an entire yard and the man only had three pennies to give her; but she knew this would buy some bread for her children, so she said, "I was glad to do it."

She talked about this difficult time in her life as if it was another person and she was telling a story. She held her head high and sat up straight

127

as she conveyed the story to me. She looked at me and smiled as she said, "I have never had a food stamp or a government check of any kind until I went on Social Security. When my children were growing up I bought a paper and they had to read to me every night. There was no television or radio in our home – just books. I could not help their growing up as poor, black children, but I could help them from growing up to be poor and ignorant children."

Ms. Lucille developed pneumonia and became very critically ill. Her family was called in. I was privileged to meet these children whom she adored. The two daughters were physicians and the two sons were attorneys.

I have to tell you that in my entire career as a Nurse, never had I witnessed such a tender, precious love for a mother than these children showed as their mother lay dying. Those big, tall, and very strong professional children kissed their mother's hand and lay in the bed with her until she died – whispering their love messages and thanking her over and over again for what she had done for them. This lady had lived a life of giving and she had raised four children who had dedicated their lives to giving as well.

What a privilege it was for me to have had the opportunity to care for such a human being. When I think of Ms. Lucille, I am ennobled and mentally empowered to do more as a Nurse – to go the extra mile to make sure the patients for whom I care receive the best possible attention. I feel knowing Ms. Lucille was one of the greatest gifts I have ever had as a Nurse. She had a direct influence on how I see older patients, especially the confused and mentally challenged. All I can say is, "Thank you Ms. Lucille for having a part in making me the successful Nurse that I am today." She could not tell you one thing about today, yesterday, last week, or last year, but she could talk in detail about her life as a young mother.

Ms. Lucille never entered the End Stage of Alzheimer's. She retained her beauty and grace until the moment she died. Her Alzheimer's took a lot of her away, but it did not take away Ms. Lucille – only death did that and in reality, not even death took away Ms. Lucille, because she lives in the hearts of everyone she met, myself among the vast number.

In Conclusion

I would like to thank all the speakers I have been privileged to listen to from the Alzheimer's Associations in Utah, New Jersey, and North Carolina. These organizations have taught me much of what I have learned as a Geriatric Nurse in relation to Alzheimer's and Dementia.

These organizations are not only available to the medical profession, but to families as well. If you need help or want more information on Alzheimer's or Dementia, go to any Nursing Home, Hospital, or Assisted Living and ask for the Alzheimer Association telephone number. They can help with finding support groups, Alzheimer's units, and Doctors. They are there for you and they want to help.

There is so much more information on Alzheimer's that I could not put in this book, but if you want to know more, go to your library or go online and you will discover a lot of valuable, helpful information at such sites as:

http://www.alz.org/aboutAD/causes.asp

If you are a caregiver of a mentally challenged patient of any kind and you feel depressed, angry, or out of control, go to a Doctor and get help. How can you care for a family member with Alzheimer's when you are not well yourself? You owe it to yourself and to your loved one.

Life is very complicated for many people. Society has placed on all of us stresses that can oftentimes create havoc in our lives, but for patients who have Alzheimer's or Dementia, life can NO longer be allowed to be complicated. It needs to be kept as simple as possible.

The everyday life for Alzheimer's/Dementia patients is broken down into simple tasks, mental stimulation as much as possible, keeping them safe from themselves and others, giving them the dignity, respect, independence, privacy, and autonomy they have earned throughout their productive years.

I have endeavored to keep this book simple for you, as a loved one or caregiver. It is an uphill battle with this disease, but fought in the correct way, everyone can come out the better. In the final months and years for Alzheimer's patients, they should be protected at all costs from those who might exploit them or inflict harm.

I often reminded my staff at meetings, "We are where they have been and they are possibly where we are going." I sometimes had family members bring in pictures of residents when they were young and I would place the photos in the middle of the table and have my staff to look at them. They talked about how beautiful the women were and how handsome the men were. I told them that all those pictures were the people they were caring for everyday. It made such an impact on my staff to see these patients as they had once been. It helped create in them a greater desire to care for and protect them with even more of a professional manner and mannerisms.

Never forget to remind yourself on a daily basis of "that" mom or dad (or other loved one) before Alzheimer's – the way he or she was – not the way he or she is. Try to picture your loved one as a captive with the disease of Alzheimer's – he or she is being held as a prisoner. They cannot get out and you cannot get in, except when occasionally the door opens. WHEN IT DOES - BE THERE FOR THEM. Walk through the door and visit with your loved one for as long as the door is open. Remember those times, cherish them, and know that the door will eventually not open at all for your loved one, but you will have precious memories. And when everything is over, the peace of mind you have will be priceless. You will know you were there for your loved one – you saw that he or she received the best care possible and you exhausted every means to give all that was required and needed to make the final months and years as normal as possible.

If you do this - In the battle with this disease you truly will come out the WINNER!

About the Author

Rebecca Jarrard, since 1972, **has lived a childhood dream of being a Nurse**. She has been involved in a variety of areas in the medical profession, such as: Home Health Nursing, Oncology, Medical Surgical, Geriatric and Orthopedic Nursing. **For the last seven years most of her work has been in the Dementia and Alzheimer's field.**

While living in Utah, Rebecca was a **"Charge Nurse"** on an Alzheimer's Unit where she observed that the overwhelming majority of caregivers did not know how to take care of the patients. They knew very little of redirection and when the residents became agitated and combative, staff members often ran from the patients; many times leaving the unit and thus leaving the residents with no supervision. There were few, to no, activities so the residents wandered aimlessly about the unit.

Upon moving to New Jersey, in 2000, Rebecca accepted a position as **Director and Wellness Nurse** on a 30-bed Alzheimer's/Dementia Unit. <u>During her 31/2-year tenure on this unit, the unit remained **deficiency free** and **recommendation free** by the State of New Jersey.</u> She assisted in the clinical training of Medication Aides and Assisted Living Administrators. The unit she worked on was chosen as one of the field sites for graduate students from the University of North Carolina to observe behavior patterns of people with

Alzheimer's and Dementia. **She also worked with a national drug company to develop a brochure for family members on "Caring For The Patient With Alzheimer's And Dementia."**

Rebecca presently resides in North Carolina with her husband, Dan.

Printed in the United States
57786LVS00001B/52-135